This
KETO DIET JOURNAL
Belongs To:

_____

Ketogenic Foods

MEATS	VEGGIES	VEGGIES	FRUITS
Beef	Avocado	Cucumber	Blackberries
Sausage	Asparagus	Chards	Cranberries
Bacon	Argula	Bell Peppers	Blueberries
Lamb	Broccoli	Green Beans	Lemon
Pork	Cauliflower	Collards	Lime
Veal	Brussel Sprouts	Mushrooms	Raspberries
Chicken/Turkey	Cabbage	Spinach	Strawberries
Eggs	Celery	Olives	Plantains (paleo)

DAIRY	CONDIMENTS	OILS & FATS	HERBS & SPICES
Cheese (all kinds)	Balsamic Vinegar	Avocado Oil	Garlic
Sour Cream	Beef/Chicken Broth	Butter	Salt & Pepper
Cream Cheese	Bonito Flakes	Coconut Butter	Oregano
Heavy Cream	Tartar Sauce (keto)	Duck Fat	Paprika
Greek Yogurt	Dijon Mustard	Lard/Ghee	Cumin
Almond Milk	Mayo	Nut Oils	Chili Pepper
Cashew Milk	Low Sugar Ketchup	Olive Oil	Basil
Coconut Cream	Pickles	Pork Rinds	Ginger

BAKING	FISH/SEAFOOD	DRINKS	MISC.
Almond Flour	Anchovy	Diet Soda (moderation)	Canned Tuna
Almond Meal	Haddock / Cod	Coffee	Pesto
Cashew Flour	Halibut	Tea	Soy Sauce
Oat Fiber	Crab/Lobster	Gatorade Zero	Aioli
Psyllium Husk	Mackerel	Protein Shake	Béarnaise
Whey Protein	Salmon	Club Soda	Vinaigrette
Flax meal	Tuna	Broth	Hot Sauce
Hazelnut Flour	Red Snapper	Coconut Water	Guacamole

NOTES:

Keto Grocery Inventory

DATE: _____

QTY	PRODUCE

QTY	MEAT & FISH

QTY	FROZEN FOODS

QTY	DAIRY

QTY	PANTRY

QTY	OTHER/MISC.

Macro Quick Reference

MACRO TRACKER

QTY	TYPE	PROTEIN	FAT	CARBS	CALS	NOTES

Keto Goals

1 USE THIS KETO JOURNAL AND DOCUMENT YOUR PROGRESS — COMPLETED ☐	**2** CHOOSE 7 KETO FRIENDLY RECIPES TO TRY — COMPLETED ☐	**3** CREATE A WEEKLY MEAL PLAN — COMPLETED ☐
4 WRITE DOWN EVERYTHING YOU EAT IN THIS PLANNER — COMPLETED ☐	**5** PURCHASE A FOOD SCALE AND SPIRALIZER — COMPLETED ☐	**6** TRY BULLET PROOF COFFEE — COMPLETED ☐
7 WEIGH YOURSELF ONCE A WEEK — COMPLETED ☐	**8** GO ALCOHOL FREE FOR ONE WEEK — COMPLETED ☐	**9** TRY A 12-HOUR INTERMITTENT FAST — COMPLETED ☐
10 CHECK AND LOG YOUR BODY MEASUREMENTS — COMPLETED ☐	**11** LIST ALL THE REASONS WHY KETO WILL WORK FOR YOU — COMPLETED ☐	**12** LEARN TO MAKE FAT BOMBS — COMPLETED ☐
13 MONITOR YOUR WATER INTAKE — COMPLETED ☐	**14** INCREASE YOUR HEALTHY FAT INTAKE — COMPLETED ☐	**15** TEST KETONE LEVELS USING STRIPS — COMPLETED ☐

KETO BEFORE *& After*

WEIGHT	WEIGHT
BMI	BMI
BODY FAT	BODY FAT
MUSCLE	MUSCLE
CHEST	CHEST
WAIST	WAIST
HIPS	HIPS
THIGHS	THIGHS
CALF	CALF
BICEP	BICEP
OTHER :	OTHER :
OTHER :	OTHER :

Weight and Measurements

Chest

Arm

Waist

Hips

Thigh

STARTING MEASUREMENTS:

WEIGHT:

LEFT ARM:

RIGHT ARM:

CHEST:

WAIST:

HIPS:

LEFT THIGH:

RIGHT THIGH:

My Journey

PERSONAL GOALS:

90 Days of Keto

Count down the next 90 days and track your progress!

STARTING WEIGHT:

DAY 90 WEIGHT:

| 1 | 2 | 3 | 4 | 5 | 6 | 7 | 8 | 9 | 10 |
LBS LOST:
INCHES LOST:

| 11 | 12 | 13 | 14 | 15 | 16 | 17 | 18 | 19 | 20 |
LBS LOST:
INCHES LOST:

| 21 | 22 | 23 | 24 | 25 | 26 | 27 | 28 | 29 | 30 |
LBS LOST:
INCHES LOST:

| 31 | 32 | 33 | 34 | 35 | 36 | 37 | 38 | 39 | 40 |
LBS LOST:
INCHES LOST:

| 41 | 42 | 43 | 44 | 45 | 46 | 47 | 48 | 49 | 50 |
LBS LOST:
INCHES LOST:

| 51 | 52 | 53 | 54 | 55 | 56 | 57 | 58 | 59 | 60 |
LBS LOST:
INCHES LOST:

| 61 | 62 | 63 | 64 | 65 | 66 | 67 | 68 | 69 | 70 |
LBS LOST:
INCHES LOST:

| 71 | 72 | 73 | 74 | 75 | 76 | 77 | 78 | 79 | 80 |
LBS LOST:
INCHES LOST:

| 81 | 82 | 83 | 84 | 85 | 86 | 87 | 88 | 89 | 90 |
LBS LOST:
INCHES LOST:

TOTAL WEIGHT LOST:

TOTAL INCHES LOST:

NOTES & REFLECTIONS:

21 DAY KETO *Challenge*

It takes just 21 days to create a healthy routine that will last a lifetime!
Let's stay in ketosis for 21 days!

START DATE	END DATE

1	2	3	4	5
6	7	8	9	10
11	12	13	14	15
16	17	18	19	20

21	NOTES

KETO GO TO *Meals*

FAVORITE KETO FRIENDLY MEALS

BREAKFAST	LUNCH	DINNER	SNACKS
BREAKFAST	LUNCH	DINNER	SNACKS
BREAKFAST	LUNCH	DINNER	SNACKS
BREAKFAST	LUNCH	DINNER	SNACKS
BREAKFAST	LUNCH	DINNER	SNACKS
BREAKFAST	LUNCH	DINNER	SNACKS
BREAKFAST	LUNCH	DINNER	SNACKS

Favorite *Keto-Friendly Foods*

KETO FRIENDLY FOODS	NET CARBS	PROTEINS	FAT

FOODS TO EAT IN MODERATION	NET CARBS	PROTEINS	FAT

KETO *Journal*

MY KETO JOURNEY *Tracker*

SLEEP TRACKER:

DATE _____

☀ RISE: _____   🌙 zzz BEDTIME: _____   💭 zᶻz SLEEP (HRS): _____

NOTES FOR THE DAY

_____

_____

_____

IN A STATE OF KETOSIS?

YES   NO   UNSURE

WATER INTAKE TRACKER

EXERCISE / WORKOUT ROUTINE

DAILY ENERGY LEVEL		
HIGH	**MEDIUM**	**LOW**

BREAKFAST

FAT: CARBS: PROTEIN: CALORIES:

LUNCH

FAT: CARBS: PROTEIN: CALORIES:

DINNER

FAT: CARBS: PROTEIN: CALORIES:

SNACKS

FAT: CARBS: PROTEIN: CALORIES:

TOP 6 PRIORITIES OF THE DAY

END OF THE DAY TOTAL OVERVIEW

CARBS	FAT	PROTEIN	CALORIES

DAILY FOOD *Journal*

FOOD TRACKER

MEAL/SNACK	NET CARBS	FAT	CAL	PROTEIN
DAILY GOAL:				
TOTAL:				

MY KETO JOURNEY *Tracker*

SLEEP TRACKER:

DATE _____

☀ RISE: _____

🌙 z z z BEDTIME: _____

💭 zᶻZ SLEEP (HRS): _____

NOTES FOR THE DAY

_____
_____
_____

IN A STATE OF KETOSIS?

YES   NO   UNSURE

WATER INTAKE TRACKER

EXERCISE / WORKOUT ROUTINE

DAILY ENERGY LEVEL

HIGH	**MEDIUM**	**LOW**

BREAKFAST

FAT: CARBS: PROTEIN: CALORIES:

LUNCH

FAT: CARBS: PROTEIN: CALORIES:

DINNER

FAT: CARBS: PROTEIN: CALORIES:

SNACKS

FAT: CARBS: PROTEIN: CALORIES:

TOP 6 PRIORITIES OF THE DAY

END OF THE DAY TOTAL OVERVIEW

CARBS	FAT	PROTEIN	CALORIES

DAILY FOOD *Journal*

FOOD TRACKER

MEAL/SNACK	NET CARBS	FAT	CAL	PROTEIN
DAILY GOAL:				
TOTAL:				

NOTES & MEAL IDEAS

MY KETO JOURNEY *Tracker*

SLEEP TRACKER:

DATE _____

☀ RISE: [ ] 🌙 BEDTIME: [ ] 💭 SLEEP (HRS): [ ]

NOTES FOR THE DAY

_____

_____

_____

EXERCISE / WORKOUT ROUTINE

IN A STATE OF KETOSIS?

YES   NO   UNSURE

WATER INTAKE TRACKER

DAILY ENERGY LEVEL		
HIGH	**MEDIUM**	**LOW**

BREAKFAST

FAT: CARBS: PROTEIN: CALORIES:

LUNCH

FAT: CARBS: PROTEIN: CALORIES:

DINNER

FAT: CARBS: PROTEIN: CALORIES:

SNACKS

FAT: CARBS: PROTEIN: CALORIES:

TOP 6 PRIORITIES OF THE DAY

○ _____

○ _____

○ _____

END OF THE DAY TOTAL OVERVIEW

CARBS	FAT	PROTEIN	CALORIES
[ ]	[ ]	[ ]	[ ]

DAILY FOOD *Journal*

FOOD TRACKER

MEAL/SNACK	NET CARBS	FAT	CAL	PROTEIN
DAILY GOAL:				
TOTAL:				

NOTES & MEAL IDEAS

MY KETO JOURNEY *Tracker*

SLEEP TRACKER:

DATE _____

☀ | RISE: | 🌙 zᶻᶻ | BEDTIME: | 💭zᶻᶻ | SLEEP (HRS):

NOTES FOR THE DAY

_____

_____

_____

EXERCISE / WORKOUT ROUTINE

TOP 6 PRIORITIES OF THE DAY

○ _____

○ _____

○ _____

IN A STATE OF KETOSIS?

YES   NO   UNSURE

WATER INTAKE TRACKER

DAILY ENERGY LEVEL		
HIGH	**MEDIUM**	**LOW**

BREAKFAST

FAT: CARBS: PROTEIN: CALORIES:

LUNCH

FAT: CARBS: PROTEIN: CALORIES:

DINNER

FAT: CARBS: PROTEIN: CALORIES:

SNACKS

FAT: CARBS: PROTEIN: CALORIES:

END OF THE DAY TOTAL OVERVIEW

CARBS	FAT	PROTEIN	CALORIES

DAILY FOOD *Journal*

FOOD TRACKER

MEAL/SNACK	NET CARBS	FAT	CAL	PROTEIN
DAILY GOAL:				
TOTAL:				

NOTES & MEAL IDEAS

MY KETO JOURNEY *Tracker*

SLEEP TRACKER:

DATE _____

RISE: | BEDTIME: | SLEEP (HRS):

NOTES FOR THE DAY

IN A STATE OF KETOSIS?

YES   NO   UNSURE

WATER INTAKE TRACKER

EXERCISE / WORKOUT ROUTINE

DAILY ENERGY LEVEL

HIGH	**MEDIUM**	**LOW**

BREAKFAST

FAT: CARBS: PROTEIN: CALORIES:

LUNCH

FAT: CARBS: PROTEIN: CALORIES:

DINNER

FAT: CARBS: PROTEIN: CALORIES:

SNACKS

FAT: CARBS: PROTEIN: CALORIES:

TOP 6 PRIORITIES OF THE DAY

END OF THE DAY TOTAL OVERVIEW

CARBS	FAT	PROTEIN	CALORIES

DAILY FOOD *Journal*

FOOD TRACKER

MEAL/SNACK	NET CARBS	FAT	CAL	PROTEIN
DAILY GOAL:				
TOTAL:				

MY KETO JOURNEY *Tracker*

SLEEP TRACKER:

DATE _____

☀ RISE: [   ] BEDTIME: [   ] SLEEP (HRS): [   ]

NOTES FOR THE DAY

_____

_____

_____

IN A STATE OF KETOSIS?

YES   NO   UNSURE

WATER INTAKE TRACKER

EXERCISE / WORKOUT ROUTINE

DAILY ENERGY LEVEL		
HIGH	**MEDIUM**	**LOW**

BREAKFAST

FAT: CARBS: PROTEIN: CALORIES:

LUNCH

FAT: CARBS: PROTEIN: CALORIES:

DINNER

FAT: CARBS: PROTEIN: CALORIES:

SNACKS

FAT: CARBS: PROTEIN: CALORIES:

TOP 6 PRIORITIES OF THE DAY

END OF THE DAY TOTAL OVERVIEW

CARBS   FAT   PROTEIN   CALORIES

[   ]   [   ]   [   ]   [   ]

DAILY FOOD *Journal*

FOOD TRACKER

MEAL/SNACK	NET CARBS	FAT	CAL	PROTEIN
DAILY GOAL:				
TOTAL:				

NOTES & MEAL IDEAS

MY KETO JOURNEY *Tracker*

SLEEP TRACKER:

DATE _____

 RISE: [____]   BEDTIME: [____]   SLEEP (HRS): [____]

NOTES FOR THE DAY

_____
_____
_____

EXERCISE / WORKOUT ROUTINE

TOP 6 PRIORITIES OF THE DAY

○ _____   ○ _____
○ _____   ○ _____
○ _____   ○ _____

IN A STATE OF KETOSIS?

YES   NO   UNSURE

WATER INTAKE TRACKER

DAILY ENERGY LEVEL		
HIGH	**MEDIUM**	**LOW**

BREAKFAST

FAT: CARBS: PROTEIN: CALORIES:

LUNCH

FAT: CARBS: PROTEIN: CALORIES:

DINNER

FAT: CARBS: PROTEIN: CALORIES:

SNACKS

FAT: CARBS: PROTEIN: CALORIES:

END OF THE DAY TOTAL OVERVIEW

CARBS	FAT	PROTEIN	CALORIES

DAILY FOOD *Journal*

FOOD TRACKER

MEAL/SNACK	NET CARBS	FAT	CAL	PROTEIN
DAILY GOAL:				
TOTAL:				

NOTES & MEAL IDEAS

MY KETO JOURNEY *Tracker*

SLEEP TRACKER:

DATE _____

☼ RISE: | BEDTIME: | SLEEP (HRS):

NOTES FOR THE DAY

_____

_____

EXERCISE / WORKOUT ROUTINE

IN A STATE OF KETOSIS?

YES   NO   UNSURE

WATER INTAKE TRACKER

DAILY ENERGY LEVEL		
HIGH	**MEDIUM**	**LOW**

BREAKFAST

FAT: CARBS: PROTEIN: CALORIES:

LUNCH

FAT: CARBS: PROTEIN: CALORIES:

DINNER

FAT: CARBS: PROTEIN: CALORIES:

SNACKS

FAT: CARBS: PROTEIN: CALORIES:

TOP 6 PRIORITIES OF THE DAY

END OF THE DAY TOTAL OVERVIEW

CARBS   FAT   PROTEIN   CALORIES

DAILY FOOD *Journal*

FOOD TRACKER

MEAL/SNACK	NET CARBS	FAT	CAL	PROTEIN
DAILY GOAL:				
TOTAL:				

NOTES & MEAL IDEAS

MY KETO JOURNEY *Tracker*

SLEEP TRACKER:

DATE _____

 RISE: _____   BEDTIME: _____   SLEEP (HRS): _____

NOTES FOR THE DAY

_____

_____

_____

EXERCISE / WORKOUT ROUTINE

TOP 6 PRIORITIES OF THE DAY

IN A STATE OF KETOSIS?

YES   NO   UNSURE

WATER INTAKE TRACKER

DAILY ENERGY LEVEL		
HIGH	**MEDIUM**	**LOW**

BREAKFAST

FAT: CARBS: PROTEIN: CALORIES:

LUNCH

FAT: CARBS: PROTEIN: CALORIES:

DINNER

FAT: CARBS: PROTEIN: CALORIES:

SNACKS

FAT: CARBS: PROTEIN: CALORIES:

END OF THE DAY TOTAL OVERVIEW

CARBS   FAT   PROTEIN   CALORIES

DAILY FOOD *Journal*

FOOD TRACKER

MEAL/SNACK	NET CARBS	FAT	CAL	PROTEIN
DAILY GOAL:				
TOTAL:				

NOTES & MEAL IDEAS

MY KETO JOURNEY *Tracker*

SLEEP TRACKER:

DATE _____

RISE: _____   BEDTIME: _____   SLEEP (HRS): _____

NOTES FOR THE DAY

_____

_____

_____

IN A STATE OF KETOSIS?

YES   NO   UNSURE

WATER INTAKE TRACKER

EXERCISE / WORKOUT ROUTINE

DAILY ENERGY LEVEL		
HIGH	**MEDIUM**	**LOW**

BREAKFAST
FAT: CARBS: PROTEIN: CALORIES:

LUNCH
FAT: CARBS: PROTEIN: CALORIES:

DINNER
FAT: CARBS: PROTEIN: CALORIES:

SNACKS
FAT: CARBS: PROTEIN: CALORIES:

TOP 6 PRIORITIES OF THE DAY

END OF THE DAY TOTAL OVERVIEW

CARBS	FAT	PROTEIN	CALORIES

DAILY FOOD *Journal*

FOOD TRACKER

MEAL/SNACK	NET CARBS	FAT	CAL	PROTEIN
DAILY GOAL:				
TOTAL:				

NOTES & MEAL IDEAS

MY KETO JOURNEY *Tracker*

SLEEP TRACKER:

DATE _____

☼ | RISE: | 🌙 z_z^z | BEDTIME: | 💭z^z^z | SLEEP (HRS):

NOTES FOR THE DAY

_____

_____

_____

IN A STATE OF KETOSIS?

YES   NO   UNSURE

WATER INTAKE TRACKER

EXERCISE / WORKOUT ROUTINE

DAILY ENERGY LEVEL		
HIGH	**MEDIUM**	**LOW**

BREAKFAST

FAT: CARBS: PROTEIN: CALORIES:

LUNCH

FAT: CARBS: PROTEIN: CALORIES:

DINNER

FAT: CARBS: PROTEIN: CALORIES:

SNACKS

FAT: CARBS: PROTEIN: CALORIES:

TOP 6 PRIORITIES OF THE DAY

END OF THE DAY TOTAL OVERVIEW

CARBS	FAT	PROTEIN	CALORIES

DAILY FOOD *Journal*

FOOD TRACKER

MEAL/SNACK	NET CARBS	FAT	CAL	PROTEIN
DAILY GOAL:				
TOTAL:				

NOTES & MEAL IDEAS

_____

_____

_____

_____

_____

_____

_____

MY KETO JOURNEY *Tracker*

SLEEP TRACKER:

DATE _____

☼ RISE: | BEDTIME: | SLEEP (HRS):

NOTES FOR THE DAY

_____
_____
_____

EXERCISE / WORKOUT ROUTINE

TOP 6 PRIORITIES OF THE DAY

IN A STATE OF KETOSIS?

YES   NO   UNSURE

WATER INTAKE TRACKER

DAILY ENERGY LEVEL		
HIGH	**MEDIUM**	**LOW**

BREAKFAST

FAT: CARBS: PROTEIN: CALORIES:

LUNCH

FAT: CARBS: PROTEIN: CALORIES:

DINNER

FAT: CARBS: PROTEIN: CALORIES:

SNACKS

FAT: CARBS: PROTEIN: CALORIES:

END OF THE DAY TOTAL OVERVIEW

CARBS   FAT   PROTEIN   CALORIES

DAILY FOOD *Journal*

FOOD TRACKER

MEAL/SNACK	NET CARBS	FAT	CAL	PROTEIN
DAILY GOAL:				
TOTAL:				

NOTES & MEAL IDEAS

MY KETO JOURNEY *Tracker*

SLEEP TRACKER:

DATE _____

 RISE: | BEDTIME: | SLEEP (HRS):

NOTES FOR THE DAY

_____
_____
_____

IN A STATE OF KETOSIS?

YES   NO   UNSURE

WATER INTAKE TRACKER

EXERCISE / WORKOUT ROUTINE

DAILY ENERGY LEVEL		
HIGH	**MEDIUM**	**LOW**

BREAKFAST

FAT: CARBS: PROTEIN: CALORIES:

LUNCH

FAT: CARBS: PROTEIN: CALORIES:

DINNER

FAT: CARBS: PROTEIN: CALORIES:

SNACKS

FAT: CARBS: PROTEIN: CALORIES:

TOP 6 PRIORITIES OF THE DAY

END OF THE DAY TOTAL OVERVIEW

CARBS	FAT	PROTEIN	CALORIES

DAILY FOOD *Journal*

FOOD TRACKER

MEAL/SNACK	NET CARBS	FAT	CAL	PROTEIN
DAILY GOAL:				
TOTAL:				

NOTES & MEAL IDEAS

MY KETO JOURNEY *Tracker*

SLEEP TRACKER:

 RISE: | BEDTIME: | SLEEP (HRS):

DATE _____

NOTES FOR THE DAY

_____
_____
_____

IN A STATE OF KETOSIS?

YES　　　NO　　　UNSURE

WATER INTAKE TRACKER

EXERCISE / WORKOUT ROUTINE

DAILY ENERGY LEVEL		
HIGH	**MEDIUM**	**LOW**

BREAKFAST

FAT:　　CARBS:　　PROTEIN:　　CALORIES:

LUNCH

FAT:　　CARBS:　　PROTEIN:　　CALORIES:

DINNER

FAT:　　CARBS:　　PROTEIN:　　CALORIES:

SNACKS

FAT:　　CARBS:　　PROTEIN:　　CALORIES:

TOP 6 PRIORITIES OF THE DAY

END OF THE DAY TOTAL OVERVIEW

CARBS　　　FAT　　　PROTEIN　　CALORIES

DAILY FOOD *Journal*

FOOD TRACKER

MEAL/SNACK	NET CARBS	FAT	CAL	PROTEIN
DAILY GOAL:				
TOTAL:				

NOTES & MEAL IDEAS

_____

_____

_____

_____

_____

_____

_____

_____

MY KETO JOURNEY *Tracker*

SLEEP TRACKER:

DATE _____

 | RISE: _____

BEDTIME: _____

 | SLEEP (HRS): _____

NOTES FOR THE DAY

_____
_____
_____

IN A STATE OF KETOSIS?

YES   NO   UNSURE

WATER INTAKE TRACKER

EXERCISE / WORKOUT ROUTINE

DAILY ENERGY LEVEL		
HIGH	**MEDIUM**	**LOW**

BREAKFAST

FAT: CARBS: PROTEIN: CALORIES:

LUNCH

FAT: CARBS: PROTEIN: CALORIES:

DINNER

FAT: CARBS: PROTEIN: CALORIES:

SNACKS

FAT: CARBS: PROTEIN: CALORIES:

TOP 6 PRIORITIES OF THE DAY

END OF THE DAY TOTAL OVERVIEW

CARBS	FAT	PROTEIN	CALORIES

DAILY FOOD *Journal*

FOOD TRACKER					NOTES & MEAL IDEAS
MEAL/SNACK	NET CARBS	FAT	CAL	PROTEIN	
	DAILY GOAL:				
	TOTAL:				

MY KETO JOURNEY *Tracker*

SLEEP TRACKER:

DATE _____

☀ RISE: [_____]　　🌙 BEDTIME: [_____]　　💤 SLEEP (HRS): [_____]

NOTES FOR THE DAY

_____
_____
_____

EXERCISE / WORKOUT ROUTINE

TOP 6 PRIORITIES OF THE DAY

○ _____　　○ _____

○ _____　　○ _____

○ _____　　○ _____

IN A STATE OF KETOSIS?

YES　　　NO　　　UNSURE

WATER INTAKE TRACKER

DAILY ENERGY LEVEL		
HIGH	**MEDIUM**	**LOW**

BREAKFAST

FAT:	CARBS:	PROTEIN:	CALORIES:

LUNCH

FAT:	CARBS:	PROTEIN:	CALORIES:

DINNER

FAT:	CARBS:	PROTEIN:	CALORIES:

SNACKS

FAT:	CARBS:	PROTEIN:	CALORIES:

END OF THE DAY TOTAL OVERVIEW

CARBS	FAT	PROTEIN	CALORIES
[ ]	[ ]	[ ]	[ ]

DAILY FOOD *Journal*

FOOD TRACKER

MEAL/SNACK	NET CARBS	FAT	CAL	PROTEIN
DAILY GOAL:				
TOTAL:				

NOTES & MEAL IDEAS

MY KETO JOURNEY *Tracker*

SLEEP TRACKER:

DATE _____

☀ RISE: _____

🌙 ᶻᵤᶻ BEDTIME: _____

💭ᶻᵤᶻ SLEEP (HRS): _____

NOTES FOR THE DAY

_____

_____

_____

IN A STATE OF KETOSIS?

YES   NO   UNSURE

WATER INTAKE TRACKER

EXERCISE / WORKOUT ROUTINE

DAILY ENERGY LEVEL		
HIGH	**MEDIUM**	**LOW**

BREAKFAST

FAT: CARBS: PROTEIN: CALORIES:

LUNCH

FAT: CARBS: PROTEIN: CALORIES:

DINNER

FAT: CARBS: PROTEIN: CALORIES:

SNACKS

FAT: CARBS: PROTEIN: CALORIES:

TOP 6 PRIORITIES OF THE DAY

END OF THE DAY TOTAL OVERVIEW

CARBS	FAT	PROTEIN	CALORIES

DAILY FOOD *Journal*

FOOD TRACKER					NOTES & MEAL IDEAS
MEAL/SNACK	NET CARBS	FAT	CAL	PROTEIN	
DAILY GOAL:					
TOTAL:					

MY KETO JOURNEY *Tracker*

SLEEP TRACKER:

DATE _____

☀ RISE: _____   🌙 zᶻᶻ BEDTIME: _____   💭zᶻᶻ SLEEP (HRS): _____

NOTES FOR THE DAY
_____
_____
_____

IN A STATE OF KETOSIS?

YES   NO   UNSURE

WATER INTAKE TRACKER

EXERCISE / WORKOUT ROUTINE

DAILY ENERGY LEVEL		
HIGH	**MEDIUM**	**LOW**

BREAKFAST

FAT: CARBS: PROTEIN: CALORIES:

LUNCH

FAT: CARBS: PROTEIN: CALORIES:

DINNER

FAT: CARBS: PROTEIN: CALORIES:

SNACKS

FAT: CARBS: PROTEIN: CALORIES:

TOP 6 PRIORITIES OF THE DAY

END OF THE DAY TOTAL OVERVIEW

CARBS	FAT	PROTEIN	CALORIES

DAILY FOOD *Journal*

FOOD TRACKER

MEAL/SNACK	NET CARBS	FAT	CAL	PROTEIN
DAILY GOAL:				
TOTAL:				

NOTES & MEAL IDEAS

MY KETO JOURNEY *Tracker*

SLEEP TRACKER:

DATE _____

☀ RISE: _____   🌙 zᶻᶻ BEDTIME: _____   💭zᶻᶻ SLEEP (HRS): _____

NOTES FOR THE DAY

_____

_____

_____

EXERCISE / WORKOUT ROUTINE

IN A STATE OF KETOSIS?

YES   NO   UNSURE

WATER INTAKE TRACKER

DAILY ENERGY LEVEL		
HIGH	**MEDIUM**	**LOW**

BREAKFAST

FAT: CARBS: PROTEIN: CALORIES:

LUNCH

FAT: CARBS: PROTEIN: CALORIES:

DINNER

FAT: CARBS: PROTEIN: CALORIES:

SNACKS

FAT: CARBS: PROTEIN: CALORIES:

TOP 6 PRIORITIES OF THE DAY

END OF THE DAY TOTAL OVERVIEW

CARBS	FAT	PROTEIN	CALORIES

DAILY FOOD *Journal*

FOOD TRACKER					NOTES & MEAL IDEAS
MEAL/SNACK	NET CARBS	FAT	CAL	PROTEIN	
DAILY GOAL:					
TOTAL:					

MY KETO JOURNEY *Tracker*

SLEEP TRACKER:

DATE _____

 RISE: _____

 BEDTIME: _____

 SLEEP (HRS): _____

NOTES FOR THE DAY

_____

_____

_____

IN A STATE OF KETOSIS?

YES   NO   UNSURE

WATER INTAKE TRACKER

EXERCISE / WORKOUT ROUTINE

DAILY ENERGY LEVEL		
HIGH	**MEDIUM**	**LOW**

BREAKFAST

FAT: CARBS: PROTEIN: CALORIES:

LUNCH

FAT: CARBS: PROTEIN: CALORIES:

DINNER

FAT: CARBS: PROTEIN: CALORIES:

SNACKS

FAT: CARBS: PROTEIN: CALORIES:

TOP 6 PRIORITIES OF THE DAY

END OF THE DAY TOTAL OVERVIEW

CARBS   FAT   PROTEIN   CALORIES

DAILY FOOD *Journal*

FOOD TRACKER

MEAL/SNACK	NET CARBS	FAT	CAL	PROTEIN
DAILY GOAL:				
TOTAL:				

NOTES & MEAL IDEAS

MY KETO JOURNEY *Tracker*

SLEEP TRACKER:

DATE _____

RISE: _____   BEDTIME: _____   SLEEP (HRS): _____

NOTES FOR THE DAY

_____

_____

_____

IN A STATE OF KETOSIS?

YES   NO   UNSURE

WATER INTAKE TRACKER

EXERCISE / WORKOUT ROUTINE

DAILY ENERGY LEVEL		
HIGH	**MEDIUM**	**LOW**

BREAKFAST

FAT: CARBS: PROTEIN: CALORIES:

LUNCH

FAT: CARBS: PROTEIN: CALORIES:

DINNER

FAT: CARBS: PROTEIN: CALORIES:

SNACKS

FAT: CARBS: PROTEIN: CALORIES:

TOP 6 PRIORITIES OF THE DAY

END OF THE DAY TOTAL OVERVIEW

CARBS   FAT   PROTEIN   CALORIES

DAILY FOOD *Journal*

FOOD TRACKER

MEAL/SNACK	NET CARBS	FAT	CAL	PROTEIN
DAILY GOAL:				
TOTAL:				

NOTES & MEAL IDEAS

MY KETO JOURNEY *Tracker*

SLEEP TRACKER:

DATE _____

RISE: _____

BEDTIME: _____

SLEEP (HRS): _____

NOTES FOR THE DAY

_____

_____

_____

EXERCISE / WORKOUT ROUTINE

TOP 6 PRIORITIES OF THE DAY

IN A STATE OF KETOSIS?

YES   NO   UNSURE

WATER INTAKE TRACKER

DAILY ENERGY LEVEL		
HIGH	**MEDIUM**	**LOW**

BREAKFAST

FAT: CARBS: PROTEIN: CALORIES:

LUNCH

FAT: CARBS: PROTEIN: CALORIES:

DINNER

FAT: CARBS: PROTEIN: CALORIES:

SNACKS

FAT: CARBS: PROTEIN: CALORIES:

END OF THE DAY TOTAL OVERVIEW

CARBS	FAT	PROTEIN	CALORIES

DAILY FOOD *Journal*

FOOD TRACKER

MEAL/SNACK	NET CARBS	FAT	CAL	PROTEIN
DAILY GOAL:				
TOTAL:				

NOTES & MEAL IDEAS

MY KETO JOURNEY *Tracker*

SLEEP TRACKER:

DATE _____

 RISE: _____   ☾ᶻᶻᶻ BEDTIME: _____   SLEEP (HRS): _____

NOTES FOR THE DAY

_____

_____

_____

IN A STATE OF KETOSIS?

YES   NO   UNSURE

WATER INTAKE TRACKER

EXERCISE / WORKOUT ROUTINE

DAILY ENERGY LEVEL		
HIGH	**MEDIUM**	**LOW**

BREAKFAST

FAT: CARBS: PROTEIN: CALORIES:

LUNCH

FAT: CARBS: PROTEIN: CALORIES:

DINNER

FAT: CARBS: PROTEIN: CALORIES:

SNACKS

FAT: CARBS: PROTEIN: CALORIES:

TOP 6 PRIORITIES OF THE DAY

_____

_____

END OF THE DAY TOTAL OVERVIEW

CARBS   FAT   PROTEIN   CALORIES

DAILY FOOD *Journal*

FOOD TRACKER

MEAL/SNACK	NET CARBS	FAT	CAL	PROTEIN
DAILY GOAL:				
TOTAL:				

NOTES & MEAL IDEAS

MY KETO JOURNEY *Tracker*

SLEEP TRACKER:

DATE _____

 RISE: | BEDTIME: | SLEEP (HRS):

NOTES FOR THE DAY

_____

_____

_____

EXERCISE / WORKOUT ROUTINE

IN A STATE OF KETOSIS?

YES   NO   UNSURE

WATER INTAKE TRACKER

DAILY ENERGY LEVEL		
HIGH	**MEDIUM**	**LOW**

BREAKFAST

FAT: CARBS: PROTEIN: CALORIES:

LUNCH

FAT: CARBS: PROTEIN: CALORIES:

DINNER

FAT: CARBS: PROTEIN: CALORIES:

SNACKS

FAT: CARBS: PROTEIN: CALORIES:

TOP 6 PRIORITIES OF THE DAY

END OF THE DAY TOTAL OVERVIEW

CARBS	FAT	PROTEIN	CALORIES

DAILY FOOD *Journal*

FOOD TRACKER

MEAL/SNACK	NET CARBS	FAT	CAL	PROTEIN
DAILY GOAL:				
TOTAL:				

NOTES & MEAL IDEAS

MY KETO JOURNEY *Tracker*

SLEEP TRACKER:

DATE _____

RISE: | BEDTIME: | SLEEP (HRS):

NOTES FOR THE DAY

_____

_____

_____

IN A STATE OF KETOSIS?

YES   NO   UNSURE

WATER INTAKE TRACKER

EXERCISE / WORKOUT ROUTINE

DAILY ENERGY LEVEL		
HIGH	**MEDIUM**	**LOW**

BREAKFAST

FAT: CARBS: PROTEIN: CALORIES:

LUNCH

FAT: CARBS: PROTEIN: CALORIES:

DINNER

FAT: CARBS: PROTEIN: CALORIES:

SNACKS

FAT: CARBS: PROTEIN: CALORIES:

TOP 6 PRIORITIES OF THE DAY

END OF THE DAY TOTAL OVERVIEW

CARBS	FAT	PROTEIN	CALORIES

DAILY FOOD *Journal*

FOOD TRACKER

MEAL/SNACK	NET CARBS	FAT	CAL	PROTEIN
DAILY GOAL:				
TOTAL:				

NOTES & MEAL IDEAS

MY KETO JOURNEY *Tracker*

SLEEP TRACKER:

DATE _____

☼ RISE: _____   🌙 z z z BEDTIME: _____   💭 zZZ SLEEP (HRS): _____

NOTES FOR THE DAY

_____

_____

_____

IN A STATE OF KETOSIS?

YES   NO   UNSURE

WATER INTAKE TRACKER

EXERCISE / WORKOUT ROUTINE

DAILY ENERGY LEVEL		
HIGH	**MEDIUM**	**LOW**

BREAKFAST

FAT: CARBS: PROTEIN: CALORIES:

LUNCH

FAT: CARBS: PROTEIN: CALORIES:

DINNER

FAT: CARBS: PROTEIN: CALORIES:

SNACKS

FAT: CARBS: PROTEIN: CALORIES:

TOP 6 PRIORITIES OF THE DAY

END OF THE DAY TOTAL OVERVIEW

CARBS   FAT   PROTEIN   CALORIES

DAILY FOOD *Journal*

FOOD TRACKER

MEAL/SNACK	NET CARBS	FAT	CAL	PROTEIN
DAILY GOAL:				
TOTAL:				

NOTES & MEAL IDEAS

MY KETO JOURNEY *Tracker*

SLEEP TRACKER:

DATE _____

RISE: | BEDTIME: | SLEEP (HRS):

NOTES FOR THE DAY

_____

_____

_____

IN A STATE OF KETOSIS?

YES   NO   UNSURE

WATER INTAKE TRACKER

EXERCISE / WORKOUT ROUTINE

DAILY ENERGY LEVEL		
HIGH	**MEDIUM**	**LOW**

BREAKFAST

FAT: CARBS: PROTEIN: CALORIES:

LUNCH

FAT: CARBS: PROTEIN: CALORIES:

DINNER

FAT: CARBS: PROTEIN: CALORIES:

SNACKS

FAT: CARBS: PROTEIN: CALORIES:

TOP 6 PRIORITIES OF THE DAY

END OF THE DAY TOTAL OVERVIEW

CARBS   FAT   PROTEIN   CALORIES

DAILY FOOD *Journal*

FOOD TRACKER

MEAL/SNACK	NET CARBS	FAT	CAL	PROTEIN
DAILY GOAL:				
TOTAL:				

NOTES & MEAL IDEAS

MY KETO JOURNEY *Tracker*

SLEEP TRACKER:

DATE _____

☀ | RISE: | 🌙 Zzz | BEDTIME: | 💭Zzz | SLEEP (HRS):

NOTES FOR THE DAY

_____
_____
_____

IN A STATE OF KETOSIS?

YES   NO   UNSURE

WATER INTAKE TRACKER

EXERCISE / WORKOUT ROUTINE

DAILY ENERGY LEVEL		
HIGH	**MEDIUM**	**LOW**

BREAKFAST

FAT: CARBS: PROTEIN: CALORIES:

LUNCH

FAT: CARBS: PROTEIN: CALORIES:

DINNER

FAT: CARBS: PROTEIN: CALORIES:

SNACKS

FAT: CARBS: PROTEIN: CALORIES:

TOP 6 PRIORITIES OF THE DAY

END OF THE DAY TOTAL OVERVIEW

CARBS	FAT	PROTEIN	CALORIES

DAILY FOOD *Journal*

FOOD TRACKER

MEAL/SNACK	NET CARBS	FAT	CAL	PROTEIN
DAILY GOAL:				
TOTAL:				

NOTES & MEAL IDEAS

MY KETO JOURNEY *Tracker*

SLEEP TRACKER:

DATE _____

☼ | RISE: | 🌙 zᶻz | BEDTIME: | 💭zᶻz | SLEEP (HRS):

NOTES FOR THE DAY

_____

_____

_____

EXERCISE / WORKOUT ROUTINE

TOP 6 PRIORITIES OF THE DAY

IN A STATE OF KETOSIS?

YES   NO   UNSURE

WATER INTAKE TRACKER

DAILY ENERGY LEVEL		
HIGH	**MEDIUM**	**LOW**

BREAKFAST

FAT: CARBS: PROTEIN: CALORIES:

LUNCH

FAT: CARBS: PROTEIN: CALORIES:

DINNER

FAT: CARBS: PROTEIN: CALORIES:

SNACKS

FAT: CARBS: PROTEIN: CALORIES:

END OF THE DAY TOTAL OVERVIEW

CARBS	FAT	PROTEIN	CALORIES

DAILY FOOD *Journal*

FOOD TRACKER

MEAL/SNACK	NET CARBS	FAT	CAL	PROTEIN
DAILY GOAL:				
TOTAL:				

NOTES & MEAL IDEAS

MY KETO JOURNEY *Tracker*

SLEEP TRACKER:

DATE _____

☀ RISE: | 🌙 zᶻᶻ BEDTIME: | 💭zᶻᶻ SLEEP (HRS):

NOTES FOR THE DAY

_____
_____
_____

EXERCISE / WORKOUT ROUTINE

TOP 6 PRIORITIES OF THE DAY

IN A STATE OF KETOSIS?

YES   NO   UNSURE

WATER INTAKE TRACKER

DAILY ENERGY LEVEL		
HIGH	**MEDIUM**	**LOW**

BREAKFAST

FAT: CARBS: PROTEIN: CALORIES:

LUNCH

FAT: CARBS: PROTEIN: CALORIES:

DINNER

FAT: CARBS: PROTEIN: CALORIES:

SNACKS

FAT: CARBS: PROTEIN: CALORIES:

END OF THE DAY TOTAL OVERVIEW

CARBS   FAT   PROTEIN   CALORIES

DAILY FOOD *Journal*

FOOD TRACKER

MEAL/SNACK	NET CARBS	FAT	CAL	PROTEIN
DAILY GOAL:				
TOTAL:				

NOTES & MEAL IDEAS

30-DAY
Progress

Weight and Measurements

Chest

Arm

Waist

Hips

Thigh

MEASUREMENTS:

WEIGHT:

LEFT ARM:

RIGHT ARM:

CHEST:

WAIST:

HIPS:

LEFT THIGH:

RIGHT THIGH:

My Journey

THOUGHTS ON MY PROGRESS:

MY KETO JOURNEY *Tracker*

SLEEP TRACKER:

DATE _____

 RISE: | BEDTIME: | SLEEP (HRS):

NOTES FOR THE DAY

_____
_____
_____

EXERCISE / WORKOUT ROUTINE

TOP 6 PRIORITIES OF THE DAY

IN A STATE OF KETOSIS?

YES   NO   UNSURE

WATER INTAKE TRACKER

DAILY ENERGY LEVEL		
HIGH	**MEDIUM**	**LOW**

BREAKFAST

FAT: CARBS: PROTEIN: CALORIES:

LUNCH

FAT: CARBS: PROTEIN: CALORIES:

DINNER

FAT: CARBS: PROTEIN: CALORIES:

SNACKS

FAT: CARBS: PROTEIN: CALORIES:

END OF THE DAY TOTAL OVERVIEW

CARBS	FAT	PROTEIN	CALORIES

DAILY FOOD *Journal*

FOOD TRACKER

MEAL/SNACK	NET CARBS	FAT	CAL	PROTEIN
DAILY GOAL:				
TOTAL:				

NOTES & MEAL IDEAS

MY KETO JOURNEY *Tracker*

SLEEP TRACKER:

DATE _____

☼ RISE: | 🌙ᶻᶻᶻ BEDTIME: | 💭ᶻᶻᶻ SLEEP (HRS):

NOTES FOR THE DAY

_____

_____

_____

EXERCISE / WORKOUT ROUTINE

TOP 6 PRIORITIES OF THE DAY

IN A STATE OF KETOSIS?

YES   NO   UNSURE

WATER INTAKE TRACKER

DAILY ENERGY LEVEL		
HIGH	**MEDIUM**	**LOW**

BREAKFAST

FAT: CARBS: PROTEIN: CALORIES:

LUNCH

FAT: CARBS: PROTEIN: CALORIES:

DINNER

FAT: CARBS: PROTEIN: CALORIES:

SNACKS

FAT: CARBS: PROTEIN: CALORIES:

END OF THE DAY TOTAL OVERVIEW

CARBS	FAT	PROTEIN	CALORIES

DAILY FOOD *Journal*

FOOD TRACKER

MEAL/SNACK	NET CARBS	FAT	CAL	PROTEIN
DAILY GOAL:				
TOTAL:				

NOTES & MEAL IDEAS

MY KETO JOURNEY *Tracker*

SLEEP TRACKER:

DATE _____

 RISE: _____

🌙 BEDTIME: _____

 SLEEP (HRS): _____

NOTES FOR THE DAY

_____

_____

_____

IN A STATE OF KETOSIS?

YES   NO   UNSURE

WATER INTAKE TRACKER

EXERCISE / WORKOUT ROUTINE

DAILY ENERGY LEVEL		
HIGH	**MEDIUM**	**LOW**

BREAKFAST

FAT: CARBS: PROTEIN: CALORIES:

LUNCH

FAT: CARBS: PROTEIN: CALORIES:

DINNER

FAT: CARBS: PROTEIN: CALORIES:

SNACKS

FAT: CARBS: PROTEIN: CALORIES:

TOP 6 PRIORITIES OF THE DAY

END OF THE DAY TOTAL OVERVIEW

CARBS	FAT	PROTEIN	CALORIES

DAILY FOOD *Journal*

FOOD TRACKER

MEAL/SNACK	NET CARBS	FAT	CAL	PROTEIN
DAILY GOAL:				
TOTAL:				

NOTES & MEAL IDEAS

MY KETO JOURNEY *Tracker*

SLEEP TRACKER:

DATE _____

☀ RISE: _____

🌙 ᶻᶻᶻ BEDTIME: _____

💭ᶻᶻᶻ SLEEP (HRS): _____

NOTES FOR THE DAY

_____

_____

_____

EXERCISE / WORKOUT ROUTINE

TOP 6 PRIORITIES OF THE DAY

○ _____   ○ _____
○ _____   ○ _____
○ _____   ○ _____

IN A STATE OF KETOSIS?

YES   NO   UNSURE

WATER INTAKE TRACKER

DAILY ENERGY LEVEL		
HIGH	**MEDIUM**	**LOW**

BREAKFAST

FAT: CARBS: PROTEIN: CALORIES:

LUNCH

FAT: CARBS: PROTEIN: CALORIES:

DINNER

FAT: CARBS: PROTEIN: CALORIES:

SNACKS

FAT: CARBS: PROTEIN: CALORIES:

END OF THE DAY TOTAL OVERVIEW

CARBS   FAT   PROTEIN   CALORIES

DAILY FOOD *Journal*

FOOD TRACKER

MEAL/SNACK	NET CARBS	FAT	CAL	PROTEIN
DAILY GOAL:				
TOTAL:				

NOTES & MEAL IDEAS

MY KETO JOURNEY *Tracker*

SLEEP TRACKER:

DATE _____

 RISE: _____

 BEDTIME: _____

 SLEEP (HRS): _____

NOTES FOR THE DAY

_____

_____

_____

EXERCISE / WORKOUT ROUTINE

TOP 6 PRIORITIES OF THE DAY

IN A STATE OF KETOSIS?

YES   NO   UNSURE

WATER INTAKE TRACKER

DAILY ENERGY LEVEL		
HIGH	**MEDIUM**	**LOW**

BREAKFAST

FAT: CARBS: PROTEIN: CALORIES:

LUNCH

FAT: CARBS: PROTEIN: CALORIES:

DINNER

FAT: CARBS: PROTEIN: CALORIES:

SNACKS

FAT: CARBS: PROTEIN: CALORIES:

END OF THE DAY TOTAL OVERVIEW

CARBS	FAT	PROTEIN	CALORIES

DAILY FOOD *Journal*

FOOD TRACKER

MEAL/SNACK	NET CARBS	FAT	CAL	PROTEIN
DAILY GOAL:				
TOTAL:				

NOTES & MEAL IDEAS

MY KETO JOURNEY *Tracker*

SLEEP TRACKER:

DATE _____

 RISE: _____   BEDTIME: _____   SLEEP (HRS): _____

NOTES FOR THE DAY

_____

_____

_____

IN A STATE OF KETOSIS?

YES   NO   UNSURE

WATER INTAKE TRACKER

EXERCISE / WORKOUT ROUTINE

DAILY ENERGY LEVEL

HIGH	MEDIUM	LOW

BREAKFAST

FAT: CARBS: PROTEIN: CALORIES:

LUNCH

FAT: CARBS: PROTEIN: CALORIES:

DINNER

FAT: CARBS: PROTEIN: CALORIES:

SNACKS

FAT: CARBS: PROTEIN: CALORIES:

TOP 6 PRIORITIES OF THE DAY

END OF THE DAY TOTAL OVERVIEW

CARBS	FAT	PROTEIN	CALORIES

DAILY FOOD *Journal*

MEAL/SNACK	NET CARBS	FAT	CAL	PROTEIN
DAILY GOAL:				
TOTAL:				

NOTES & MEAL IDEAS

MY KETO JOURNEY *Tracker*

SLEEP TRACKER:

DATE _____

 RISE: _____   BEDTIME: _____   SLEEP (HRS): _____

NOTES FOR THE DAY

_____

_____

_____

EXERCISE / WORKOUT ROUTINE

TOP 6 PRIORITIES OF THE DAY

⊙ _____   ⊙ _____

⊙ _____   ⊙ _____

⊙ _____   ⊙ _____

IN A STATE OF KETOSIS?

YES   NO   UNSURE

WATER INTAKE TRACKER

DAILY ENERGY LEVEL		
HIGH	**MEDIUM**	**LOW**

BREAKFAST

FAT: CARBS: PROTEIN: CALORIES:

LUNCH

FAT: CARBS: PROTEIN: CALORIES:

DINNER

FAT: CARBS: PROTEIN: CALORIES:

SNACKS

FAT: CARBS: PROTEIN: CALORIES:

END OF THE DAY TOTAL OVERVIEW

CARBS	FAT	PROTEIN	CALORIES

DAILY FOOD *Journal*

FOOD TRACKER

MEAL/SNACK	NET CARBS	FAT	CAL	PROTEIN
DAILY GOAL:				
TOTAL:				

NOTES & MEAL IDEAS

MY KETO JOURNEY *Tracker*

SLEEP TRACKER:

DATE _____

 RISE: | BEDTIME: | SLEEP (HRS):

NOTES FOR THE DAY

_____
_____
_____
_____

IN A STATE OF KETOSIS?

YES   NO   UNSURE

WATER INTAKE TRACKER

EXERCISE / WORKOUT ROUTINE

DAILY ENERGY LEVEL		
HIGH	**MEDIUM**	**LOW**

BREAKFAST

FAT: CARBS: PROTEIN: CALORIES:

LUNCH

FAT: CARBS: PROTEIN: CALORIES:

DINNER

FAT: CARBS: PROTEIN: CALORIES:

SNACKS

FAT: CARBS: PROTEIN: CALORIES:

TOP 6 PRIORITIES OF THE DAY

END OF THE DAY TOTAL OVERVIEW

CARBS	FAT	PROTEIN	CALORIES

DAILY FOOD *Journal*

FOOD TRACKER

MEAL/SNACK	NET CARBS	FAT	CAL	PROTEIN
DAILY GOAL:				
TOTAL:				

NOTES & MEAL IDEAS

MY KETO JOURNEY *Tracker*

SLEEP TRACKER:

DATE _____

☼ RISE: | 🌙 zzz BEDTIME: | 💭zzz SLEEP (HRS):

NOTES FOR THE DAY

_____
_____
_____

IN A STATE OF KETOSIS?

YES   NO   UNSURE

WATER INTAKE TRACKER

EXERCISE / WORKOUT ROUTINE

DAILY ENERGY LEVEL		
HIGH	**MEDIUM**	**LOW**

BREAKFAST

FAT: CARBS: PROTEIN: CALORIES:

LUNCH

FAT: CARBS: PROTEIN: CALORIES:

DINNER

FAT: CARBS: PROTEIN: CALORIES:

SNACKS

FAT: CARBS: PROTEIN: CALORIES:

TOP 6 PRIORITIES OF THE DAY

END OF THE DAY TOTAL OVERVIEW

CARBS   FAT   PROTEIN   CALORIES

DAILY FOOD *Journal*

FOOD TRACKER

MEAL/SNACK	NET CARBS	FAT	CAL	PROTEIN
DAILY GOAL:				
TOTAL:				

NOTES & MEAL IDEAS

MY KETO JOURNEY *Tracker*

SLEEP TRACKER:

DATE _____

☼ | RISE: | 🌙 zzz | BEDTIME: | 💭zᶻz | SLEEP (HRS):

NOTES FOR THE DAY

_____

_____

_____

IN A STATE OF KETOSIS?

YES   NO   UNSURE

WATER INTAKE TRACKER

EXERCISE / WORKOUT ROUTINE

DAILY ENERGY LEVEL		
HIGH	**MEDIUM**	**LOW**

BREAKFAST

FAT: CARBS: PROTEIN: CALORIES:

LUNCH

FAT: CARBS: PROTEIN: CALORIES:

DINNER

FAT: CARBS: PROTEIN: CALORIES:

SNACKS

FAT: CARBS: PROTEIN: CALORIES:

TOP 6 PRIORITIES OF THE DAY

END OF THE DAY TOTAL OVERVIEW

CARBS	FAT	PROTEIN	CALORIES

DAILY FOOD *Journal*

FOOD TRACKER

MEAL/SNACK	NET CARBS	FAT	CAL	PROTEIN
DAILY GOAL:				
TOTAL:				

NOTES & MEAL IDEAS

MY KETO JOURNEY *Tracker*

SLEEP TRACKER:

DATE _____

☀ | RISE: | 🌙 zzZ | BEDTIME: | 💭zᶻz | SLEEP (HRS):

NOTES FOR THE DAY

_____
_____
_____

IN A STATE OF KETOSIS?

YES   NO   UNSURE

WATER INTAKE TRACKER

EXERCISE / WORKOUT ROUTINE

DAILY ENERGY LEVEL		
HIGH	**MEDIUM**	**LOW**

BREAKFAST

FAT: CARBS: PROTEIN: CALORIES:

LUNCH

FAT: CARBS: PROTEIN: CALORIES:

DINNER

FAT: CARBS: PROTEIN: CALORIES:

SNACKS

FAT: CARBS: PROTEIN: CALORIES:

TOP 6 PRIORITIES OF THE DAY

END OF THE DAY TOTAL OVERVIEW

CARBS	FAT	PROTEIN	CALORIES

DAILY FOOD *Journal*

FOOD TRACKER

MEAL/SNACK	NET CARBS	FAT	CAL	PROTEIN
DAILY GOAL:				
TOTAL:				

NOTES & MEAL IDEAS

MY KETO JOURNEY *Tracker*

SLEEP TRACKER:

DATE _____

☼ RISE: _____

🌙 zzz BEDTIME: _____

💭zᶻZ SLEEP (HRS): _____

NOTES FOR THE DAY

_____

_____

_____

IN A STATE OF KETOSIS?

YES   NO   UNSURE

WATER INTAKE TRACKER

EXERCISE / WORKOUT ROUTINE

DAILY ENERGY LEVEL		
HIGH	**MEDIUM**	**LOW**

BREAKFAST

FAT: CARBS: PROTEIN: CALORIES:

LUNCH

FAT: CARBS: PROTEIN: CALORIES:

DINNER

FAT: CARBS: PROTEIN: CALORIES:

SNACKS

FAT: CARBS: PROTEIN: CALORIES:

TOP 6 PRIORITIES OF THE DAY

END OF THE DAY TOTAL OVERVIEW

CARBS	FAT	PROTEIN	CALORIES

DAILY FOOD *Journal*

FOOD TRACKER

MEAL/SNACK	NET CARBS	FAT	CAL	PROTEIN
DAILY GOAL:				
TOTAL:				

NOTES & MEAL IDEAS

MY KETO JOURNEY *Tracker*

SLEEP TRACKER:

DATE _____

☀ RISE: _____   BEDTIME: _____   SLEEP (HRS): _____

NOTES FOR THE DAY

_____
_____
_____

IN A STATE OF KETOSIS?

YES   NO   UNSURE

WATER INTAKE TRACKER

EXERCISE / WORKOUT ROUTINE

DAILY ENERGY LEVEL		
HIGH	**MEDIUM**	**LOW**

BREAKFAST

FAT: CARBS: PROTEIN: CALORIES:

LUNCH

FAT: CARBS: PROTEIN: CALORIES:

DINNER

FAT: CARBS: PROTEIN: CALORIES:

SNACKS

FAT: CARBS: PROTEIN: CALORIES:

TOP 6 PRIORITIES OF THE DAY

_____
_____
_____

END OF THE DAY TOTAL OVERVIEW

CARBS   FAT   PROTEIN   CALORIES

DAILY FOOD *Journal*

FOOD TRACKER

MEAL/SNACK	NET CARBS	FAT	CAL	PROTEIN
DAILY GOAL:				
TOTAL:				

NOTES & MEAL IDEAS

MY KETO JOURNEY *Tracker*

SLEEP TRACKER:

DATE _____

☀ RISE: _____   ☽ zzz BEDTIME: _____   💭 zᶻz SLEEP (HRS): _____

NOTES FOR THE DAY
_____
_____
_____

EXERCISE / WORKOUT ROUTINE

IN A STATE OF KETOSIS?

YES   NO   UNSURE

WATER INTAKE TRACKER

DAILY ENERGY LEVEL		
HIGH	**MEDIUM**	**LOW**

BREAKFAST

FAT: CARBS: PROTEIN: CALORIES:

LUNCH

FAT: CARBS: PROTEIN: CALORIES:

DINNER

FAT: CARBS: PROTEIN: CALORIES:

SNACKS

FAT: CARBS: PROTEIN: CALORIES:

TOP 6 PRIORITIES OF THE DAY

END OF THE DAY TOTAL OVERVIEW

CARBS	FAT	PROTEIN	CALORIES

DAILY FOOD *Journal*

FOOD TRACKER

MEAL/SNACK	NET CARBS	FAT	CAL	PROTEIN
DAILY GOAL:				
TOTAL:				

NOTES & MEAL IDEAS

MY KETO JOURNEY *Tracker*

SLEEP TRACKER:

DATE _____

 RISE: | BEDTIME: | SLEEP (HRS):

NOTES FOR THE DAY

_____
_____
_____

EXERCISE / WORKOUT ROUTINE

TOP 6 PRIORITIES OF THE DAY

IN A STATE OF KETOSIS?

YES   NO   UNSURE

WATER INTAKE TRACKER

DAILY ENERGY LEVEL		
HIGH	**MEDIUM**	**LOW**

BREAKFAST
FAT: CARBS: PROTEIN: CALORIES:

LUNCH
FAT: CARBS: PROTEIN: CALORIES:

DINNER
FAT: CARBS: PROTEIN: CALORIES:

SNACKS
FAT: CARBS: PROTEIN: CALORIES:

END OF THE DAY TOTAL OVERVIEW

CARBS	FAT	PROTEIN	CALORIES

DAILY FOOD *Journal*

FOOD TRACKER

MEAL/SNACK	NET CARBS	FAT	CAL	PROTEIN
DAILY GOAL:				
TOTAL:				

MY KETO JOURNEY *Tracker*

SLEEP TRACKER:

DATE _____

☼ | RISE: | 🌙 zᶻᶻ | BEDTIME: | 💭zᶻᶻ | SLEEP (HRS): |

NOTES FOR THE DAY

_____

_____

_____

IN A STATE OF KETOSIS?

YES   NO   UNSURE

WATER INTAKE TRACKER

EXERCISE / WORKOUT ROUTINE

DAILY ENERGY LEVEL

HIGH	**MEDIUM**	**LOW**

BREAKFAST

FAT: CARBS: PROTEIN: CALORIES:

LUNCH

FAT: CARBS: PROTEIN: CALORIES:

DINNER

FAT: CARBS: PROTEIN: CALORIES:

SNACKS

FAT: CARBS: PROTEIN: CALORIES:

TOP 6 PRIORITIES OF THE DAY

END OF THE DAY TOTAL OVERVIEW

CARBS	FAT	PROTEIN	CALORIES

DAILY FOOD *Journal*

MEAL/SNACK	NET CARBS	FAT	CAL	PROTEIN
DAILY GOAL:				
TOTAL:				

MY KETO JOURNEY *Tracker*

SLEEP TRACKER:

DATE _____

RISE: _____

BEDTIME: _____

SLEEP (HRS): _____

NOTES FOR THE DAY

_____

_____

_____

IN A STATE OF KETOSIS?

YES   NO   UNSURE

WATER INTAKE TRACKER

EXERCISE / WORKOUT ROUTINE

DAILY ENERGY LEVEL

HIGH	MEDIUM	LOW

BREAKFAST

FAT: CARBS: PROTEIN: CALORIES:

LUNCH

FAT: CARBS: PROTEIN: CALORIES:

DINNER

FAT: CARBS: PROTEIN: CALORIES:

SNACKS

FAT: CARBS: PROTEIN: CALORIES:

TOP 6 PRIORITIES OF THE DAY

END OF THE DAY TOTAL OVERVIEW

CARBS   FAT   PROTEIN   CALORIES

DAILY FOOD *Journal*

FOOD TRACKER

MEAL/SNACK	NET CARBS	FAT	CAL	PROTEIN
DAILY GOAL:				
TOTAL:				

NOTES & MEAL IDEAS

MY KETO JOURNEY *Tracker*

SLEEP TRACKER:

DATE _____

 | RISE: | | BEDTIME: | | SLEEP (HRS): |

NOTES FOR THE DAY

_____

_____

_____

EXERCISE / WORKOUT ROUTINE

TOP 6 PRIORITIES OF THE DAY

IN A STATE OF KETOSIS?

YES   NO   UNSURE

WATER INTAKE TRACKER

DAILY ENERGY LEVEL		
HIGH	**MEDIUM**	**LOW**

BREAKFAST

FAT: CARBS: PROTEIN: CALORIES:

LUNCH

FAT: CARBS: PROTEIN: CALORIES:

DINNER

FAT: CARBS: PROTEIN: CALORIES:

SNACKS

FAT: CARBS: PROTEIN: CALORIES:

END OF THE DAY TOTAL OVERVIEW

CARBS	FAT	PROTEIN	CALORIES

DAILY FOOD *Journal*

FOOD TRACKER

MEAL/SNACK	NET CARBS	FAT	CAL	PROTEIN
DAILY GOAL:				
TOTAL:				

NOTES & MEAL IDEAS

MY KETO JOURNEY *Tracker*

SLEEP TRACKER:

DATE _____

 RISE: _____   BEDTIME: _____   SLEEP (HRS): _____

NOTES FOR THE DAY

_____
_____
_____

IN A STATE OF KETOSIS?

YES   NO   UNSURE

WATER INTAKE TRACKER

EXERCISE / WORKOUT ROUTINE

DAILY ENERGY LEVEL		
HIGH	**MEDIUM**	**LOW**

BREAKFAST

FAT: CARBS: PROTEIN: CALORIES:

LUNCH

FAT: CARBS: PROTEIN: CALORIES:

DINNER

FAT: CARBS: PROTEIN: CALORIES:

SNACKS

FAT: CARBS: PROTEIN: CALORIES:

TOP 6 PRIORITIES OF THE DAY

END OF THE DAY TOTAL OVERVIEW

CARBS	FAT	PROTEIN	CALORIES

DAILY FOOD *Journal*

FOOD TRACKER

MEAL/SNACK	NET CARBS	FAT	CAL	PROTEIN
DAILY GOAL:				
TOTAL:				

MY KETO JOURNEY *Tracker*

SLEEP TRACKER:

DATE _____

☀ | RISE: | 🌙ᶻᶻᶻ | BEDTIME: | 💭ᶻᶻᶻ | SLEEP (HRS):

NOTES FOR THE DAY

_____

_____

_____

EXERCISE / WORKOUT ROUTINE

TOP 6 PRIORITIES OF THE DAY

IN A STATE OF KETOSIS?

YES   NO   UNSURE

WATER INTAKE TRACKER

DAILY ENERGY LEVEL		
HIGH	**MEDIUM**	**LOW**

BREAKFAST

FAT: CARBS: PROTEIN: CALORIES:

LUNCH

FAT: CARBS: PROTEIN: CALORIES:

DINNER

FAT: CARBS: PROTEIN: CALORIES:

SNACKS

FAT: CARBS: PROTEIN: CALORIES:

END OF THE DAY TOTAL OVERVIEW

CARBS	FAT	PROTEIN	CALORIES

DAILY FOOD *Journal*

FOOD TRACKER

MEAL/SNACK	NET CARBS	FAT	CAL	PROTEIN
DAILY GOAL:				
TOTAL:				

NOTES & MEAL IDEAS

MY KETO JOURNEY *Tracker*

SLEEP TRACKER:

DATE _____

☀ RISE: _____   🌙 z z z BEDTIME: _____   💭 z z z SLEEP (HRS): _____

NOTES FOR THE DAY

_____

_____

_____

IN A STATE OF KETOSIS?

YES   NO   UNSURE

WATER INTAKE TRACKER

EXERCISE / WORKOUT ROUTINE

DAILY ENERGY LEVEL		
HIGH	**MEDIUM**	**LOW**

BREAKFAST

FAT: CARBS: PROTEIN: CALORIES:

LUNCH

FAT: CARBS: PROTEIN: CALORIES:

DINNER

FAT: CARBS: PROTEIN: CALORIES:

SNACKS

FAT: CARBS: PROTEIN: CALORIES:

TOP 6 PRIORITIES OF THE DAY

END OF THE DAY TOTAL OVERVIEW

CARBS	FAT	PROTEIN	CALORIES

DAILY FOOD *Journal*

FOOD TRACKER

MEAL/SNACK	NET CARBS	FAT	CAL	PROTEIN
DAILY GOAL:				
TOTAL:				

NOTES & MEAL IDEAS

MY KETO JOURNEY *Tracker*

SLEEP TRACKER:

DATE _____

☼ RISE: | 🌙 zzz BEDTIME: | 💭 zᶻz SLEEP (HRS): |

NOTES FOR THE DAY

_____

_____

_____

IN A STATE OF KETOSIS?

YES   NO   UNSURE

WATER INTAKE TRACKER

EXERCISE / WORKOUT ROUTINE

DAILY ENERGY LEVEL

HIGH   **MEDIUM**   **LOW**

BREAKFAST

FAT: CARBS: PROTEIN: CALORIES:

LUNCH

FAT: CARBS: PROTEIN: CALORIES:

DINNER

FAT: CARBS: PROTEIN: CALORIES:

SNACKS

FAT: CARBS: PROTEIN: CALORIES:

TOP 6 PRIORITIES OF THE DAY

_____

_____

_____

END OF THE DAY TOTAL OVERVIEW

CARBS   FAT   PROTEIN   CALORIES

DAILY FOOD *Journal*

MEAL/SNACK	NET CARBS	FAT	CAL	PROTEIN
DAILY GOAL:				
TOTAL:				

MY KETO JOURNEY *Tracker*

SLEEP TRACKER:

DATE _____

 RISE: _____

 BEDTIME: _____

SLEEP (HRS): _____

NOTES FOR THE DAY
_____
_____
_____

IN A STATE OF KETOSIS?

YES   NO   UNSURE

WATER INTAKE TRACKER

EXERCISE / WORKOUT ROUTINE

DAILY ENERGY LEVEL

HIGH	**MEDIUM**	**LOW**

BREAKFAST

FAT: CARBS: PROTEIN: CALORIES:

LUNCH

FAT: CARBS: PROTEIN: CALORIES:

DINNER

FAT: CARBS: PROTEIN: CALORIES:

SNACKS

FAT: CARBS: PROTEIN: CALORIES:

TOP 6 PRIORITIES OF THE DAY

END OF THE DAY TOTAL OVERVIEW

CARBS	FAT	PROTEIN	CALORIES

DAILY FOOD *Journal*

FOOD TRACKER

MEAL/SNACK	NET CARBS	FAT	CAL	PROTEIN
DAILY GOAL:				
TOTAL:				

NOTES & MEAL IDEAS

MY KETO JOURNEY *Tracker*

SLEEP TRACKER:

DATE _____

 RISE: [   ]   BEDTIME: [   ]   SLEEP (HRS): [   ]

NOTES FOR THE DAY

_____

_____

_____

IN A STATE OF KETOSIS?

YES   NO   UNSURE

WATER INTAKE TRACKER

EXERCISE / WORKOUT ROUTINE

[   ]

DAILY ENERGY LEVEL		
HIGH	**MEDIUM**	**LOW**

BREAKFAST

FAT: CARBS: PROTEIN: CALORIES:

LUNCH

FAT: CARBS: PROTEIN: CALORIES:

DINNER

FAT: CARBS: PROTEIN: CALORIES:

SNACKS

FAT: CARBS: PROTEIN: CALORIES:

TOP 6 PRIORITIES OF THE DAY

END OF THE DAY TOTAL OVERVIEW

CARBS   FAT   PROTEIN   CALORIES

DAILY FOOD *Journal*

FOOD TRACKER

MEAL/SNACK	NET CARBS	FAT	CAL	PROTEIN
DAILY GOAL:				
TOTAL:				

NOTES & MEAL IDEAS

MY KETO JOURNEY *Tracker*

SLEEP TRACKER:

DATE _____

☀ RISE: | 🌙 BEDTIME: | 💭 SLEEP (HRS):

NOTES FOR THE DAY

_____
_____
_____

EXERCISE / WORKOUT ROUTINE

IN A STATE OF KETOSIS?

YES   NO   UNSURE

WATER INTAKE TRACKER

DAILY ENERGY LEVEL		
HIGH	**MEDIUM**	**LOW**

BREAKFAST

FAT: CARBS: PROTEIN: CALORIES:

LUNCH

FAT: CARBS: PROTEIN: CALORIES:

DINNER

FAT: CARBS: PROTEIN: CALORIES:

SNACKS

FAT: CARBS: PROTEIN: CALORIES:

TOP 6 PRIORITIES OF THE DAY

END OF THE DAY TOTAL OVERVIEW

CARBS	FAT	PROTEIN	CALORIES

DAILY FOOD *Journal*

FOOD TRACKER

MEAL/SNACK	NET CARBS	FAT	CAL	PROTEIN
DAILY GOAL:				
TOTAL:				

NOTES & MEAL IDEAS

MY KETO JOURNEY *Tracker*

SLEEP TRACKER:

DATE _____

☼ RISE: _____   🌙 ᶻᶻᶻ BEDTIME: _____   💭ᶻᶻᶻ SLEEP (HRS): _____

NOTES FOR THE DAY

_____

_____

_____

EXERCISE / WORKOUT ROUTINE

TOP 6 PRIORITIES OF THE DAY

IN A STATE OF KETOSIS?

YES   NO   UNSURE

WATER INTAKE TRACKER

DAILY ENERGY LEVEL		
HIGH	**MEDIUM**	**LOW**

BREAKFAST

FAT: CARBS: PROTEIN: CALORIES:

LUNCH

FAT: CARBS: PROTEIN: CALORIES:

DINNER

FAT: CARBS: PROTEIN: CALORIES:

SNACKS

FAT: CARBS: PROTEIN: CALORIES:

END OF THE DAY TOTAL OVERVIEW

CARBS	FAT	PROTEIN	CALORIES

DAILY FOOD *Journal*

FOOD TRACKER

MEAL/SNACK	NET CARBS	FAT	CAL	PROTEIN
DAILY GOAL:				
TOTAL:				

MY KETO JOURNEY *Tracker*

SLEEP TRACKER:

DATE _____

☼ RISE: _____ 🌙 zzz BEDTIME: _____ 💭zᶻZ SLEEP (HRS): _____

NOTES FOR THE DAY

_____

_____

_____

IN A STATE OF KETOSIS?

YES   NO   UNSURE

WATER INTAKE TRACKER

EXERCISE / WORKOUT ROUTINE

DAILY ENERGY LEVEL		
HIGH	**MEDIUM**	**LOW**

BREAKFAST

FAT: CARBS: PROTEIN: CALORIES:

LUNCH

FAT: CARBS: PROTEIN: CALORIES:

DINNER

FAT: CARBS: PROTEIN: CALORIES:

SNACKS

FAT: CARBS: PROTEIN: CALORIES:

TOP 6 PRIORITIES OF THE DAY

END OF THE DAY TOTAL OVERVIEW

CARBS	FAT	PROTEIN	CALORIES

DAILY FOOD *Journal*

FOOD TRACKER

MEAL/SNACK	NET CARBS	FAT	CAL	PROTEIN
DAILY GOAL:				
TOTAL:				

NOTES & MEAL IDEAS

MY KETO JOURNEY *Tracker*

SLEEP TRACKER:

DATE _____

RISE: | BEDTIME: | SLEEP (HRS):

NOTES FOR THE DAY

_____

_____

_____

EXERCISE / WORKOUT ROUTINE

TOP 6 PRIORITIES OF THE DAY

IN A STATE OF KETOSIS?

YES   NO   UNSURE

WATER INTAKE TRACKER

DAILY ENERGY LEVEL		
HIGH	**MEDIUM**	**LOW**

BREAKFAST

FAT: CARBS: PROTEIN: CALORIES:

LUNCH

FAT: CARBS: PROTEIN: CALORIES:

DINNER

FAT: CARBS: PROTEIN: CALORIES:

SNACKS

FAT: CARBS: PROTEIN: CALORIES:

END OF THE DAY TOTAL OVERVIEW

CARBS	FAT	PROTEIN	CALORIES

DAILY FOOD *Journal*

FOOD TRACKER

MEAL/SNACK	NET CARBS	FAT	CAL	PROTEIN
DAILY GOAL:				
TOTAL:				

MY KETO JOURNEY *Tracker*

SLEEP TRACKER:

DATE _____

 RISE: _____   🌙 zᵤᶻ BEDTIME: _____   💭zᶻᶻ SLEEP (HRS): _____

NOTES FOR THE DAY

_____

_____

_____

EXERCISE / WORKOUT ROUTINE

TOP 6 PRIORITIES OF THE DAY

○ _____   ○ _____

○ _____   ○ _____

○ _____   ○ _____

IN A STATE OF KETOSIS?

YES   NO   UNSURE

WATER INTAKE TRACKER

DAILY ENERGY LEVEL		
HIGH	**MEDIUM**	**LOW**

BREAKFAST

FAT: CARBS: PROTEIN: CALORIES:

LUNCH

FAT: CARBS: PROTEIN: CALORIES:

DINNER

FAT: CARBS: PROTEIN: CALORIES:

SNACKS

FAT: CARBS: PROTEIN: CALORIES:

END OF THE DAY TOTAL OVERVIEW

CARBS   FAT   PROTEIN   CALORIES

DAILY FOOD *Journal*

FOOD TRACKER

MEAL/SNACK	NET CARBS	FAT	CAL	PROTEIN
DAILY GOAL:				
TOTAL:				

NOTES & MEAL IDEAS

MY KETO JOURNEY *Tracker*

SLEEP TRACKER:

DATE _____

☀ | RISE: | 🌙 zzz | BEDTIME: | 💭zᶻZ | SLEEP (HRS):

NOTES FOR THE DAY

_____
_____
_____

IN A STATE OF KETOSIS?

YES   NO   UNSURE

WATER INTAKE TRACKER

EXERCISE / WORKOUT ROUTINE

DAILY ENERGY LEVEL

HIGH	**MEDIUM**	**LOW**

BREAKFAST

FAT: CARBS: PROTEIN: CALORIES:

LUNCH

FAT: CARBS: PROTEIN: CALORIES:

DINNER

FAT: CARBS: PROTEIN: CALORIES:

SNACKS

FAT: CARBS: PROTEIN: CALORIES:

TOP 6 PRIORITIES OF THE DAY

END OF THE DAY TOTAL OVERVIEW

CARBS	FAT	PROTEIN	CALORIES

DAILY FOOD *Journal*

FOOD TRACKER

MEAL/SNACK	NET CARBS	FAT	CAL	PROTEIN
DAILY GOAL:				
TOTAL:				

NOTES & MEAL IDEAS

60-DAY
Progress

Weight and Measurements

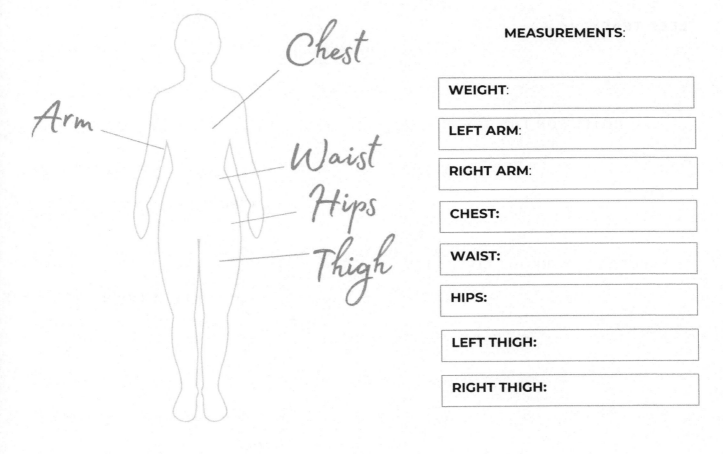

MEASUREMENTS:

WEIGHT:	
LEFT ARM:	
RIGHT ARM:	
CHEST:	
WAIST:	
HIPS:	
LEFT THIGH:	
RIGHT THIGH:	

My Journey

THOUGHTS ON MY PROGRESS:

MY KETO JOURNEY *Tracker*

SLEEP TRACKER:

RISE: _____   BEDTIME: _____   SLEEP (HRS): _____

NOTES FOR THE DAY

_____

_____

_____

IN A STATE OF KETOSIS?

YES   NO   UNSURE

WATER INTAKE TRACKER

EXERCISE / WORKOUT ROUTINE

DAILY ENERGY LEVEL

HIGH   **MEDIUM**   **LOW**

BREAKFAST

FAT: CARBS: PROTEIN: CALORIES:

LUNCH

FAT: CARBS: PROTEIN: CALORIES:

DINNER

FAT: CARBS: PROTEIN: CALORIES:

SNACKS

FAT: CARBS: PROTEIN: CALORIES:

TOP 6 PRIORITIES OF THE DAY

END OF THE DAY TOTAL OVERVIEW

CARBS   FAT   PROTEIN   CALORIES

DAILY FOOD *Journal*

FOOD TRACKER

MEAL/SNACK	NET CARBS	FAT	CAL	PROTEIN
DAILY GOAL:				
TOTAL:				

NOTES & MEAL IDEAS

MY KETO JOURNEY *Tracker*

SLEEP TRACKER:

DATE _____

RISE: _____ BEDTIME: _____ SLEEP (HRS): _____

NOTES FOR THE DAY	IN A STATE OF KETOSIS?

_____

_____

_____

YES   NO   UNSURE

WATER INTAKE TRACKER

EXERCISE / WORKOUT ROUTINE

DAILY ENERGY LEVEL		
HIGH	**MEDIUM**	**LOW**

BREAKFAST

FAT: CARBS: PROTEIN: CALORIES:

LUNCH

FAT: CARBS: PROTEIN: CALORIES:

DINNER

FAT: CARBS: PROTEIN: CALORIES:

SNACKS

FAT: CARBS: PROTEIN: CALORIES:

TOP 6 PRIORITIES OF THE DAY

END OF THE DAY TOTAL OVERVIEW

CARBS   FAT   PROTEIN   CALORIES

DAILY FOOD *Journal*

FOOD TRACKER

MEAL/SNACK	NET CARBS	FAT	CAL	PROTEIN
DAILY GOAL:				
TOTAL:				

NOTES & MEAL IDEAS

MY KETO JOURNEY *Tracker*

SLEEP TRACKER:

 RISE: BEDTIME: SLEEP (HRS):

DATE _____

NOTES FOR THE DAY

_____

_____

_____

IN A STATE OF KETOSIS?

YES   NO   UNSURE

WATER INTAKE TRACKER

EXERCISE / WORKOUT ROUTINE

DAILY ENERGY LEVEL		
HIGH	**MEDIUM**	**LOW**

BREAKFAST

FAT: CARBS: PROTEIN: CALORIES:

LUNCH

FAT: CARBS: PROTEIN: CALORIES:

DINNER

FAT: CARBS: PROTEIN: CALORIES:

SNACKS

FAT: CARBS: PROTEIN: CALORIES:

TOP 6 PRIORITIES OF THE DAY

END OF THE DAY TOTAL OVERVIEW

CARBS   FAT   PROTEIN   CALORIES

DAILY FOOD *Journal*

FOOD TRACKER

MEAL/SNACK	NET CARBS	FAT	CAL	PROTEIN
DAILY GOAL:				
TOTAL:				

NOTES & MEAL IDEAS

MY KETO JOURNEY *Tracker*

SLEEP TRACKER:

DATE _____

☀ RISE: [_____] 🌙 BEDTIME: [_____] 💭 SLEEP (HRS): [_____]

NOTES FOR THE DAY

_____
_____
_____

EXERCISE / WORKOUT ROUTINE

TOP 6 PRIORITIES OF THE DAY

❀ _____ ❀ _____
❀ _____ ❀ _____
❀ _____ ❀ _____

IN A STATE OF KETOSIS?

YES   NO   UNSURE

WATER INTAKE TRACKER

DAILY ENERGY LEVEL		
HIGH	**MEDIUM**	**LOW**

BREAKFAST

FAT: CARBS: PROTEIN: CALORIES:

LUNCH

FAT: CARBS: PROTEIN: CALORIES:

DINNER

FAT: CARBS: PROTEIN: CALORIES:

SNACKS

FAT: CARBS: PROTEIN: CALORIES:

END OF THE DAY TOTAL OVERVIEW

CARBS	FAT	PROTEIN	CALORIES
[ ]	[ ]	[ ]	[ ]

DAILY FOOD *Journal*

FOOD TRACKER

MEAL/SNACK	NET CARBS	FAT	CAL	PROTEIN
DAILY GOAL:				
TOTAL:				

NOTES & MEAL IDEAS

MY KETO JOURNEY *Tracker*

SLEEP TRACKER:

DATE _____

| RISE: | BEDTIME: | SLEEP (HRS): |

NOTES FOR THE DAY

_____
_____
_____

IN A STATE OF KETOSIS?

YES   NO   UNSURE

WATER INTAKE TRACKER

EXERCISE / WORKOUT ROUTINE

DAILY ENERGY LEVEL		
HIGH	**MEDIUM**	**LOW**

BREAKFAST

FAT: CARBS: PROTEIN: CALORIES:

LUNCH

FAT: CARBS: PROTEIN: CALORIES:

DINNER

FAT: CARBS: PROTEIN: CALORIES:

SNACKS

FAT: CARBS: PROTEIN: CALORIES:

TOP 6 PRIORITIES OF THE DAY

END OF THE DAY TOTAL OVERVIEW

CARBS	FAT	PROTEIN	CALORIES

DAILY FOOD *Journal*

FOOD TRACKER

MEAL/SNACK	NET CARBS	FAT	CAL	PROTEIN
DAILY GOAL:				
TOTAL:				

NOTES & MEAL IDEAS

MY KETO JOURNEY *Tracker*

SLEEP TRACKER:

 RISE: 🌙 BEDTIME: SLEEP (HRS):

DATE _____

NOTES FOR THE DAY

_____

_____

_____

EXERCISE / WORKOUT ROUTINE

TOP 6 PRIORITIES OF THE DAY

IN A STATE OF KETOSIS?

YES   NO   UNSURE

WATER INTAKE TRACKER

DAILY ENERGY LEVEL		
HIGH	**MEDIUM**	**LOW**

BREAKFAST

FAT: CARBS: PROTEIN: CALORIES:

LUNCH

FAT: CARBS: PROTEIN: CALORIES:

DINNER

FAT: CARBS: PROTEIN: CALORIES:

SNACKS

FAT: CARBS: PROTEIN: CALORIES:

END OF THE DAY TOTAL OVERVIEW

CARBS	FAT	PROTEIN	CALORIES

DAILY FOOD *Journal*

FOOD TRACKER

MEAL/SNACK	NET CARBS	FAT	CAL	PROTEIN
DAILY GOAL:				
TOTAL:				

NOTES & MEAL IDEAS

MY KETO JOURNEY *Tracker*

SLEEP TRACKER:

RISE: [_____]   BEDTIME: [_____]   SLEEP (HRS): [_____]

NOTES FOR THE DAY

_____
_____
_____

EXERCISE / WORKOUT ROUTINE

TOP 6 PRIORITIES OF THE DAY

IN A STATE OF KETOSIS?

YES   NO   UNSURE

WATER INTAKE TRACKER

DAILY ENERGY LEVEL

HIGH   **MEDIUM**   **LOW**

BREAKFAST

FAT: CARBS: PROTEIN: CALORIES:

LUNCH

FAT: CARBS: PROTEIN: CALORIES:

DINNER

FAT: CARBS: PROTEIN: CALORIES:

SNACKS

FAT: CARBS: PROTEIN: CALORIES:

END OF THE DAY TOTAL OVERVIEW

CARBS   FAT   PROTEIN   CALORIES

DAILY FOOD *Journal*

FOOD TRACKER

MEAL/SNACK	NET CARBS	FAT	CAL	PROTEIN
DAILY GOAL:				
TOTAL:				

MY KETO JOURNEY *Tracker*

SLEEP TRACKER:

DATE _____

☀ RISE: _____   🌙 zᶻᶻ BEDTIME: _____   💭 SLEEP (HRS): _____

NOTES FOR THE DAY

_____

_____

_____

IN A STATE OF KETOSIS?

YES   NO   UNSURE

WATER INTAKE TRACKER

EXERCISE / WORKOUT ROUTINE

DAILY ENERGY LEVEL		
HIGH	**MEDIUM**	**LOW**

BREAKFAST

FAT: CARBS: PROTEIN: CALORIES:

LUNCH

FAT: CARBS: PROTEIN: CALORIES:

DINNER

FAT: CARBS: PROTEIN: CALORIES:

SNACKS

FAT: CARBS: PROTEIN: CALORIES:

TOP 6 PRIORITIES OF THE DAY

END OF THE DAY TOTAL OVERVIEW

CARBS   FAT   PROTEIN   CALORIES

DAILY FOOD *Journal*

FOOD TRACKER

MEAL/SNACK	NET CARBS	FAT	CAL	PROTEIN
DAILY GOAL:				
TOTAL:				

NOTES & MEAL IDEAS

MY KETO JOURNEY *Tracker*

SLEEP TRACKER:

DATE _____

 RISE: [   ]   BEDTIME: [   ]   SLEEP (HRS): [   ]

NOTES FOR THE DAY

_____

_____

_____

IN A STATE OF KETOSIS?

YES   NO   UNSURE

WATER INTAKE TRACKER

EXERCISE / WORKOUT ROUTINE

DAILY ENERGY LEVEL		
HIGH	**MEDIUM**	**LOW**

BREAKFAST

FAT: CARBS: PROTEIN: CALORIES:

LUNCH

FAT: CARBS: PROTEIN: CALORIES:

DINNER

FAT: CARBS: PROTEIN: CALORIES:

SNACKS

FAT: CARBS: PROTEIN: CALORIES:

TOP 6 PRIORITIES OF THE DAY

○ _____   ○ _____

○ _____   ○ _____

○ _____   ○ _____

END OF THE DAY TOTAL OVERVIEW

CARBS   FAT   PROTEIN   CALORIES

DAILY FOOD *Journal*

FOOD TRACKER

MEAL/SNACK	NET CARBS	FAT	CAL	PROTEIN
DAILY GOAL:				
TOTAL:				

NOTES & MEAL IDEAS

MY KETO JOURNEY *Tracker*

SLEEP TRACKER:

DATE _____

 RISE:

 BEDTIME:

 SLEEP (HRS):

NOTES FOR THE DAY

_____

_____

_____

IN A STATE OF KETOSIS?

YES   NO   UNSURE

WATER INTAKE TRACKER

EXERCISE / WORKOUT ROUTINE

DAILY ENERGY LEVEL		
HIGH	**MEDIUM**	**LOW**

BREAKFAST

FAT: CARBS: PROTEIN: CALORIES:

LUNCH

FAT: CARBS: PROTEIN: CALORIES:

DINNER

FAT: CARBS: PROTEIN: CALORIES:

SNACKS

FAT: CARBS: PROTEIN: CALORIES:

TOP 6 PRIORITIES OF THE DAY

- _____   - _____
- _____   - _____
- _____   - _____

END OF THE DAY TOTAL OVERVIEW

CARBS   FAT   PROTEIN   CALORIES

DAILY FOOD *Journal*

FOOD TRACKER

MEAL/SNACK	NET CARBS	FAT	CAL	PROTEIN
DAILY GOAL:				
TOTAL:				

NOTES & MEAL IDEAS

MY KETO JOURNEY *Tracker*

SLEEP TRACKER:

DATE _____

 RISE: _____

BEDTIME: _____

 SLEEP (HRS): _____

NOTES FOR THE DAY

_____
_____
_____

EXERCISE / WORKOUT ROUTINE

IN A STATE OF KETOSIS?

YES   NO   UNSURE

WATER INTAKE TRACKER

DAILY ENERGY LEVEL

HIGH	**MEDIUM**	**LOW**

BREAKFAST

FAT: CARBS: PROTEIN: CALORIES:

LUNCH

FAT: CARBS: PROTEIN: CALORIES:

DINNER

FAT: CARBS: PROTEIN: CALORIES:

SNACKS

FAT: CARBS: PROTEIN: CALORIES:

TOP 6 PRIORITIES OF THE DAY

END OF THE DAY TOTAL OVERVIEW

CARBS	FAT	PROTEIN	CALORIES

DAILY FOOD *Journal*

FOOD TRACKER

MEAL/SNACK	NET CARBS	FAT	CAL	PROTEIN
DAILY GOAL:				
TOTAL:				

NOTES & MEAL IDEAS

MY KETO JOURNEY *Tracker*

SLEEP TRACKER:

DATE _____

☀ RISE: _____   🌙 BEDTIME: _____   💭 SLEEP (HRS): _____

NOTES FOR THE DAY

_____

_____

_____

EXERCISE / WORKOUT ROUTINE

TOP 6 PRIORITIES OF THE DAY

IN A STATE OF KETOSIS?

YES   NO   UNSURE

WATER INTAKE TRACKER

DAILY ENERGY LEVEL		
HIGH	**MEDIUM**	**LOW**

BREAKFAST

FAT: CARBS: PROTEIN: CALORIES:

LUNCH

FAT: CARBS: PROTEIN: CALORIES:

DINNER

FAT: CARBS: PROTEIN: CALORIES:

SNACKS

FAT: CARBS: PROTEIN: CALORIES:

END OF THE DAY TOTAL OVERVIEW

CARBS	FAT	PROTEIN	CALORIES

DAILY FOOD *Journal*

FOOD TRACKER

MEAL/SNACK	NET CARBS	FAT	CAL	PROTEIN
DAILY GOAL:				
TOTAL:				

NOTES & MEAL IDEAS

MY KETO JOURNEY *Tracker*

SLEEP TRACKER:

DATE _____

☀ | RISE: | 🌙 | BEDTIME: | 💭 | SLEEP (HRS):

NOTES FOR THE DAY

_____

_____

_____

EXERCISE / WORKOUT ROUTINE

TOP 6 PRIORITIES OF THE DAY

IN A STATE OF KETOSIS?

YES   NO   UNSURE

WATER INTAKE TRACKER

DAILY ENERGY LEVEL		
HIGH	**MEDIUM**	**LOW**

BREAKFAST

FAT: CARBS: PROTEIN: CALORIES:

LUNCH

FAT: CARBS: PROTEIN: CALORIES:

DINNER

FAT: CARBS: PROTEIN: CALORIES:

SNACKS

FAT: CARBS: PROTEIN: CALORIES:

END OF THE DAY TOTAL OVERVIEW

CARBS   FAT   PROTEIN   CALORIES

DAILY FOOD *Journal*

FOOD TRACKER

MEAL/SNACK	NET CARBS	FAT	CAL	PROTEIN
DAILY GOAL:				
TOTAL:				

NOTES & MEAL IDEAS

MY KETO JOURNEY *Tracker*

SLEEP TRACKER:

DATE _____

 RISE: _____

 BEDTIME: _____

 SLEEP (HRS): _____

NOTES FOR THE DAY

_____
_____
_____

IN A STATE OF KETOSIS?

YES   NO   UNSURE

WATER INTAKE TRACKER

EXERCISE / WORKOUT ROUTINE

DAILY ENERGY LEVEL		
HIGH	**MEDIUM**	**LOW**

BREAKFAST

FAT: CARBS: PROTEIN: CALORIES:

LUNCH

FAT: CARBS: PROTEIN: CALORIES:

DINNER

FAT: CARBS: PROTEIN: CALORIES:

SNACKS

FAT: CARBS: PROTEIN: CALORIES:

TOP 6 PRIORITIES OF THE DAY

END OF THE DAY TOTAL OVERVIEW

CARBS   FAT   PROTEIN   CALORIES

DAILY FOOD *Journal*

MEAL/SNACK	NET CARBS	FAT	CAL	PROTEIN
DAILY GOAL:				
TOTAL:				

NOTES & MEAL IDEAS

MY KETO JOURNEY *Tracker*

SLEEP TRACKER:

DATE _____

☀ | RISE: | 🌙 zzz | BEDTIME: | 💭zᶻZ | SLEEP (HRS):

NOTES FOR THE DAY

_____

_____

_____

IN A STATE OF KETOSIS?

YES   NO   UNSURE

WATER INTAKE TRACKER

EXERCISE / WORKOUT ROUTINE

DAILY ENERGY LEVEL

HIGH	**MEDIUM**	**LOW**

BREAKFAST

FAT: CARBS: PROTEIN: CALORIES:

LUNCH

FAT: CARBS: PROTEIN: CALORIES:

DINNER

FAT: CARBS: PROTEIN: CALORIES:

SNACKS

FAT: CARBS: PROTEIN: CALORIES:

TOP 6 PRIORITIES OF THE DAY

END OF THE DAY TOTAL OVERVIEW

CARBS	FAT	PROTEIN	CALORIES

DAILY FOOD *Journal*

FOOD TRACKER

MEAL/SNACK	NET CARBS	FAT	CAL	PROTEIN
DAILY GOAL:				
TOTAL:				

NOTES & MEAL IDEAS

MY KETO JOURNEY *Tracker*

SLEEP TRACKER:

DATE _____

 RISE: | BEDTIME: | SLEEP (HRS):

NOTES FOR THE DAY

_____

_____

_____

EXERCISE / WORKOUT ROUTINE

TOP 6 PRIORITIES OF THE DAY

○ _____   ○ _____

○ _____   ○ _____

○ _____   ○ _____

IN A STATE OF KETOSIS?

YES   NO   UNSURE

WATER INTAKE TRACKER

DAILY ENERGY LEVEL		
HIGH	**MEDIUM**	**LOW**

BREAKFAST

FAT: CARBS: PROTEIN: CALORIES:

LUNCH

FAT: CARBS: PROTEIN: CALORIES:

DINNER

FAT: CARBS: PROTEIN: CALORIES:

SNACKS

FAT: CARBS: PROTEIN: CALORIES:

END OF THE DAY TOTAL OVERVIEW

CARBS	FAT	PROTEIN	CALORIES

DAILY FOOD *Journal*

FOOD TRACKER

MEAL/SNACK	NET CARBS	FAT	CAL	PROTEIN
DAILY GOAL:				
TOTAL:				

NOTES & MEAL IDEAS

MY KETO JOURNEY *Tracker*

SLEEP TRACKER:

DATE _____

☀ RISE: | 🌙 BEDTIME: | 💤 SLEEP (HRS):

NOTES FOR THE DAY

_____
_____
_____

IN A STATE OF KETOSIS?

YES   NO   UNSURE

WATER INTAKE TRACKER

EXERCISE / WORKOUT ROUTINE

DAILY ENERGY LEVEL		
HIGH	**MEDIUM**	**LOW**

BREAKFAST

FAT: CARBS: PROTEIN: CALORIES:

LUNCH

FAT: CARBS: PROTEIN: CALORIES:

DINNER

FAT: CARBS: PROTEIN: CALORIES:

SNACKS

FAT: CARBS: PROTEIN: CALORIES:

TOP 6 PRIORITIES OF THE DAY

END OF THE DAY TOTAL OVERVIEW

CARBS   FAT   PROTEIN   CALORIES

DAILY FOOD *Journal*

FOOD TRACKER

MEAL/SNACK	NET CARBS	FAT	CAL	PROTEIN
DAILY GOAL:				
TOTAL:				

MY KETO JOURNEY *Tracker*

SLEEP TRACKER:

DATE _____

RISE: _____

BEDTIME: _____

SLEEP (HRS): _____

NOTES FOR THE DAY

_____

_____

_____

EXERCISE / WORKOUT ROUTINE

TOP 6 PRIORITIES OF THE DAY

IN A STATE OF KETOSIS?

YES   NO   UNSURE

WATER INTAKE TRACKER

DAILY ENERGY LEVEL		
HIGH	**MEDIUM**	**LOW**

BREAKFAST

FAT: CARBS: PROTEIN: CALORIES:

LUNCH

FAT: CARBS: PROTEIN: CALORIES:

DINNER

FAT: CARBS: PROTEIN: CALORIES:

SNACKS

FAT: CARBS: PROTEIN: CALORIES:

END OF THE DAY TOTAL OVERVIEW

CARBS   FAT   PROTEIN   CALORIES

DAILY FOOD *Journal*

FOOD TRACKER

MEAL/SNACK	NET CARBS	FAT	CAL	PROTEIN
DAILY GOAL:				
TOTAL:				

NOTES & MEAL IDEAS

MY KETO JOURNEY *Tracker*

SLEEP TRACKER:

DATE _____

 RISE: _____   BEDTIME: _____   SLEEP (HRS): _____

NOTES FOR THE DAY

_____

_____

_____

IN A STATE OF KETOSIS?

YES   NO   UNSURE

WATER INTAKE TRACKER

EXERCISE / WORKOUT ROUTINE

DAILY ENERGY LEVEL		
HIGH	**MEDIUM**	**LOW**

BREAKFAST

FAT: CARBS: PROTEIN: CALORIES:

LUNCH

FAT: CARBS: PROTEIN: CALORIES:

DINNER

FAT: CARBS: PROTEIN: CALORIES:

SNACKS

FAT: CARBS: PROTEIN: CALORIES:

TOP 6 PRIORITIES OF THE DAY

END OF THE DAY TOTAL OVERVIEW

CARBS	FAT	PROTEIN	CALORIES

DAILY FOOD *Journal*

FOOD TRACKER

MEAL/SNACK	NET CARBS	FAT	CAL	PROTEIN
DAILY GOAL:				
TOTAL:				

NOTES & MEAL IDEAS

MY KETO JOURNEY *Tracker*

SLEEP TRACKER:

DATE _____

☀ RISE: _____   🌙 zzz BEDTIME: _____   💭 zzz SLEEP (HRS): _____

NOTES FOR THE DAY

_____
_____
_____

EXERCISE / WORKOUT ROUTINE

TOP 6 PRIORITIES OF THE DAY

⚬ _____   ⚬ _____
⚬ _____   ⚬ _____
⚬ _____   ⚬ _____

IN A STATE OF KETOSIS?

YES   NO   UNSURE

WATER INTAKE TRACKER

DAILY ENERGY LEVEL		
HIGH	**MEDIUM**	**LOW**

BREAKFAST

FAT: CARBS: PROTEIN: CALORIES:

LUNCH

FAT: CARBS: PROTEIN: CALORIES:

DINNER

FAT: CARBS: PROTEIN: CALORIES:

SNACKS

FAT: CARBS: PROTEIN: CALORIES:

END OF THE DAY TOTAL OVERVIEW

CARBS   FAT   PROTEIN   CALORIES

DAILY FOOD *Journal*

FOOD TRACKER

MEAL/SNACK	NET CARBS	FAT	CAL	PROTEIN
DAILY GOAL:				
TOTAL:				

NOTES & MEAL IDEAS

MY KETO JOURNEY *Tracker*

SLEEP TRACKER:

DATE _____

☀ RISE: [   ]   🌙 BEDTIME: [   ]   💤 SLEEP (HRS): [   ]

NOTES FOR THE DAY

_____

_____

_____

EXERCISE / WORKOUT ROUTINE

TOP 6 PRIORITIES OF THE DAY

IN A STATE OF KETOSIS?

YES   NO   UNSURE

WATER INTAKE TRACKER

DAILY ENERGY LEVEL		
HIGH	**MEDIUM**	**LOW**

BREAKFAST

FAT: CARBS: PROTEIN: CALORIES:

LUNCH

FAT: CARBS: PROTEIN: CALORIES:

DINNER

FAT: CARBS: PROTEIN: CALORIES:

SNACKS

FAT: CARBS: PROTEIN: CALORIES:

END OF THE DAY TOTAL OVERVIEW

CARBS   FAT   PROTEIN   CALORIES

[   ]   [   ]   [   ]

DAILY FOOD *Journal*

FOOD TRACKER

MEAL/SNACK	NET CARBS	FAT	CAL	PROTEIN
DAILY GOAL:				
TOTAL:				

NOTES & MEAL IDEAS

_____

_____

_____

_____

_____

_____

_____

MY KETO JOURNEY *Tracker*

SLEEP TRACKER:

DATE _____

| ☀ RISE: | 🌙 zᶻᶻ BEDTIME: | 💭 zᶻᶻ SLEEP (HRS): |

NOTES FOR THE DAY

_____

_____

_____

EXERCISE / WORKOUT ROUTINE

TOP 6 PRIORITIES OF THE DAY

○ _____   ○ _____

○ _____   ○ _____

○ _____   ○ _____

IN A STATE OF KETOSIS?

YES   NO   UNSURE

WATER INTAKE TRACKER

DAILY ENERGY LEVEL

| **HIGH** | **MEDIUM** | **LOW** |

BREAKFAST

| FAT: | CARBS: | PROTEIN: | CALORIES: |

LUNCH

| FAT: | CARBS: | PROTEIN: | CALORIES: |

DINNER

| FAT: | CARBS: | PROTEIN: | CALORIES: |

SNACKS

| FAT: | CARBS: | PROTEIN: | CALORIES: |

END OF THE DAY TOTAL OVERVIEW

CARBS	FAT	PROTEIN	CALORIES

DAILY FOOD *Journal*

FOOD TRACKER

MEAL/SNACK	NET CARBS	FAT	CAL	PROTEIN
DAILY GOAL:				
TOTAL:				

NOTES & MEAL IDEAS

MY KETO JOURNEY *Tracker*

SLEEP TRACKER:

DATE _____

RISE: _____

BEDTIME: _____

SLEEP (HRS): _____

NOTES FOR THE DAY

_____
_____
_____

IN A STATE OF KETOSIS?

YES   NO   UNSURE

WATER INTAKE TRACKER

EXERCISE / WORKOUT ROUTINE

DAILY ENERGY LEVEL		
HIGH	**MEDIUM**	**LOW**

BREAKFAST

FAT: CARBS: PROTEIN: CALORIES:

LUNCH

FAT: CARBS: PROTEIN: CALORIES:

DINNER

FAT: CARBS: PROTEIN: CALORIES:

SNACKS

FAT: CARBS: PROTEIN: CALORIES:

TOP 6 PRIORITIES OF THE DAY

END OF THE DAY TOTAL OVERVIEW

CARBS	FAT	PROTEIN	CALORIES

DAILY FOOD *Journal*

FOOD TRACKER

MEAL/SNACK	NET CARBS	FAT	CAL	PROTEIN
DAILY GOAL:				
TOTAL:				

NOTES & MEAL IDEAS

MY KETO JOURNEY *Tracker*

SLEEP TRACKER:

DATE _____

☀ | RISE: _____ | 🌙 zᶻᶻ | BEDTIME: _____ | 💭zᶻᶻ | SLEEP (HRS): _____

NOTES FOR THE DAY

_____

_____

_____

EXERCISE / WORKOUT ROUTINE

IN A STATE OF KETOSIS?

YES   NO   UNSURE

WATER INTAKE TRACKER

DAILY ENERGY LEVEL

HIGH	**MEDIUM**	**LOW**

BREAKFAST

FAT: CARBS: PROTEIN: CALORIES:

LUNCH

FAT: CARBS: PROTEIN: CALORIES:

DINNER

FAT: CARBS: PROTEIN: CALORIES:

SNACKS

FAT: CARBS: PROTEIN: CALORIES:

TOP 6 PRIORITIES OF THE DAY

END OF THE DAY TOTAL OVERVIEW

CARBS	FAT	PROTEIN	CALORIES

DAILY FOOD *Journal*

FOOD TRACKER

MEAL/SNACK	NET CARBS	FAT	CAL	PROTEIN
DAILY GOAL:				
TOTAL:				

NOTES & MEAL IDEAS

MY KETO JOURNEY *Tracker*

SLEEP TRACKER:

DATE _____

☀ | RISE: | 🌙 zᶻᶻ | BEDTIME: | 💭zᶻᶻ | SLEEP (HRS):

NOTES FOR THE DAY

_____
_____
_____

IN A STATE OF KETOSIS?

YES   NO   UNSURE

WATER INTAKE TRACKER

EXERCISE / WORKOUT ROUTINE

DAILY ENERGY LEVEL		
HIGH	**MEDIUM**	**LOW**

BREAKFAST

FAT: CARBS: PROTEIN: CALORIES:

LUNCH

FAT: CARBS: PROTEIN: CALORIES:

DINNER

FAT: CARBS: PROTEIN: CALORIES:

SNACKS

FAT: CARBS: PROTEIN: CALORIES:

TOP 6 PRIORITIES OF THE DAY

○ _____   ○ _____
○ _____   ○ _____
○ _____   ○ _____

END OF THE DAY TOTAL OVERVIEW

CARBS   FAT   PROTEIN   CALORIES

DAILY FOOD *Journal*

FOOD TRACKER

MEAL/SNACK	NET CARBS	FAT	CAL	PROTEIN
DAILY GOAL:				
TOTAL:				

NOTES & MEAL IDEAS

MY KETO JOURNEY *Tracker*

SLEEP TRACKER:

DATE _____

☀ RISE: _____   🌙 BEDTIME: _____   💤 SLEEP (HRS): _____

NOTES FOR THE DAY

_____

_____

_____

EXERCISE / WORKOUT ROUTINE

TOP 6 PRIORITIES OF THE DAY

○ _____   ○ _____

○ _____   ○ _____

○ _____   ○ _____

IN A STATE OF KETOSIS?

YES   NO   UNSURE

WATER INTAKE TRACKER

DAILY ENERGY LEVEL		
HIGH	**MEDIUM**	**LOW**

BREAKFAST

FAT: CARBS: PROTEIN: CALORIES:

LUNCH

FAT: CARBS: PROTEIN: CALORIES:

DINNER

FAT: CARBS: PROTEIN: CALORIES:

SNACKS

FAT: CARBS: PROTEIN: CALORIES:

END OF THE DAY TOTAL OVERVIEW

CARBS	FAT	PROTEIN	CALORIES
☐	☐	☐	☐

DAILY FOOD *Journal*

FOOD TRACKER

MEAL/SNACK	NET CARBS	FAT	CAL	PROTEIN
DAILY GOAL:				
TOTAL:				

NOTES & MEAL IDEAS

MY KETO JOURNEY *Tracker*

SLEEP TRACKER:

DATE _____

☀ RISE: [_____] 🌙 BEDTIME: [_____] 💤 SLEEP (HRS): [_____]

NOTES FOR THE DAY

_____

_____

_____

IN A STATE OF KETOSIS?

YES   NO   UNSURE

WATER INTAKE TRACKER

EXERCISE / WORKOUT ROUTINE

DAILY ENERGY LEVEL		
HIGH	**MEDIUM**	**LOW**

BREAKFAST

FAT: CARBS: PROTEIN: CALORIES:

LUNCH

FAT: CARBS: PROTEIN: CALORIES:

DINNER

FAT: CARBS: PROTEIN: CALORIES:

SNACKS

FAT: CARBS: PROTEIN: CALORIES:

TOP 6 PRIORITIES OF THE DAY

○ _____   ○ _____

○ _____   ○ _____

○ _____   ○ _____

END OF THE DAY TOTAL OVERVIEW

CARBS   FAT   PROTEIN   CALORIES

[____]   [____]   [____]   [____]

DAILY FOOD *Journal*

FOOD TRACKER

MEAL/SNACK	NET CARBS	FAT	CAL	PROTEIN

	DAILY GOAL:			
	TOTAL:			

NOTES & MEAL IDEAS

MY KETO JOURNEY *Tracker*

SLEEP TRACKER:

DATE _____

 RISE: [   ]   BEDTIME: [   ]   SLEEP (HRS): [   ]

NOTES FOR THE DAY

_____
_____
_____

IN A STATE OF KETOSIS?

YES   NO   UNSURE

WATER INTAKE TRACKER

EXERCISE / WORKOUT ROUTINE

DAILY ENERGY LEVEL		
HIGH	**MEDIUM**	**LOW**

BREAKFAST

FAT: CARBS: PROTEIN: CALORIES:

LUNCH

FAT: CARBS: PROTEIN: CALORIES:

DINNER

FAT: CARBS: PROTEIN: CALORIES:

SNACKS

FAT: CARBS: PROTEIN: CALORIES:

TOP 6 PRIORITIES OF THE DAY

○ _____   ○ _____
○ _____   ○ _____
○ _____   ○ _____

END OF THE DAY TOTAL OVERVIEW

CARBS   FAT   PROTEIN   CALORIES

[ ]   [ ]   [ ]   [ ]

DAILY FOOD *Journal*

FOOD TRACKER

MEAL/SNACK	NET CARBS	FAT	CAL	PROTEIN
DAILY GOAL:				
TOTAL:				

NOTES & MEAL IDEAS

MY KETO JOURNEY *Tracker*

SLEEP TRACKER:

DATE _____

☼ | RISE: | 🌙 | BEDTIME: | 💤 | SLEEP (HRS):

NOTES FOR THE DAY

_____

_____

_____

EXERCISE / WORKOUT ROUTINE

IN A STATE OF KETOSIS?

YES   NO   UNSURE

WATER INTAKE TRACKER

DAILY ENERGY LEVEL		
HIGH	**MEDIUM**	**LOW**

BREAKFAST

FAT: CARBS: PROTEIN: CALORIES:

LUNCH

FAT: CARBS: PROTEIN: CALORIES:

DINNER

FAT: CARBS: PROTEIN: CALORIES:

SNACKS

FAT: CARBS: PROTEIN: CALORIES:

TOP 6 PRIORITIES OF THE DAY

○ _____   ○ _____

○ _____   ○ _____

○ _____   ○ _____

END OF THE DAY TOTAL OVERVIEW

CARBS   FAT   PROTEIN   CALORIES

□   □   □   □

DAILY FOOD *Journal*

FOOD TRACKER

MEAL/SNACK	NET CARBS	FAT	CAL	PROTEIN
DAILY GOAL:				
TOTAL:				

NOTES & MEAL IDEAS

MY KETO JOURNEY *Tracker*

SLEEP TRACKER:

DATE _____

 RISE: | BEDTIME: | SLEEP (HRS):

NOTES FOR THE DAY

_____

_____

_____

IN A STATE OF KETOSIS?

YES   NO   UNSURE

WATER INTAKE TRACKER

EXERCISE / WORKOUT ROUTINE

DAILY ENERGY LEVEL		
HIGH	**MEDIUM**	**LOW**

BREAKFAST

FAT: CARBS: PROTEIN: CALORIES:

LUNCH

FAT: CARBS: PROTEIN: CALORIES:

DINNER

FAT: CARBS: PROTEIN: CALORIES:

SNACKS

FAT: CARBS: PROTEIN: CALORIES:

TOP 6 PRIORITIES OF THE DAY

END OF THE DAY TOTAL OVERVIEW

CARBS	FAT	PROTEIN	CALORIES

DAILY FOOD *Journal*

FOOD TRACKER

MEAL/SNACK	NET CARBS	FAT	CAL	PROTEIN
DAILY GOAL:				
TOTAL:				

NOTES & MEAL IDEAS

90-DAY

You Did It!

Progress

Weight and Measurements

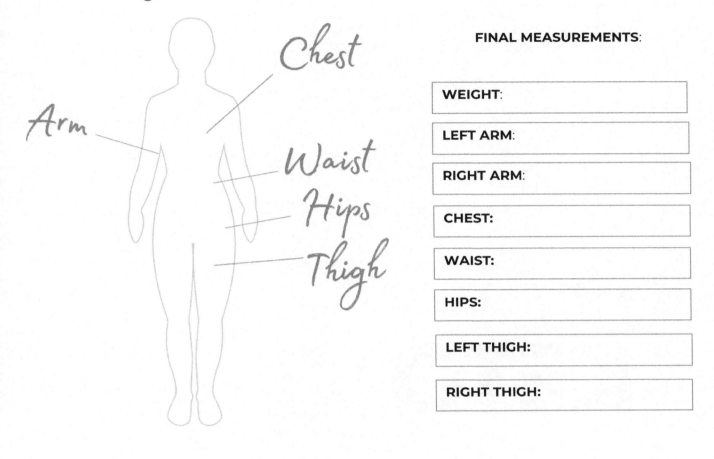

Arm

Chest

Waist

Hips

Thigh

FINAL MEASUREMENTS:

WEIGHT:

LEFT ARM:

RIGHT ARM:

CHEST:

WAIST:

HIPS:

LEFT THIGH:

RIGHT THIGH:

My Journey

THOUGHTS ON MY KETO JOURNEY:

My KETO Recipes

KETO *Recipe*

RECIPE NAME:

_____

Keto	Low Carb	Paleo	Vegetarian	Vegan	Dairy Free	Gluten Free
☐	☐	☐	☐	☐	☐	☐

QTY	INGREDIENTS

RECIPE INSTRUCTIONS

NOTES & RECIPE REVIEW

Serves	
Prep Time	
Cook Time	
Tools	
Temp	

	Carbs	Fat	Protein	Cals
Total				

KETO *Recipe*

RECIPE NAME:

_____

	Keto	Low Carb	Paleo	Vegetarian	Vegan	Dairy Free	Gluten Free
	☐	☐	☐	☐	☐	☐	☐

QTY	INGREDIENTS	RECIPE INSTRUCTIONS

NOTES & RECIPE REVIEW

Serves	
Prep Time	
Cook Time	
Tools	
Temp	

	Carbs	Fat	Protein	Cals
Total				

KETO *Recipe*

RECIPE NAME:

_____

Keto	Low Carb	Paleo	Vegetarian	Vegan	Dairy Free	Gluten Free
☐	☐	☐	☐	☐	☐	☐

QTY	INGREDIENTS

RECIPE INSTRUCTIONS

NOTES & RECIPE REVIEW

Serves	
Prep Time	
Cook Time	
Tools	
Temp	

	Carbs	Fat	Protein	Cals
Total				

KETO *Recipe*

RECIPE NAME:

_____

	Keto	Low Carb	Paleo	Vegetarian	Vegan	Dairy Free	Gluten Free
	☐	☐	☐	☐	☐	☐	☐

QTY	INGREDIENTS	RECIPE INSTRUCTIONS

NOTES & RECIPE REVIEW

Serves	
Prep Time	
Cook Time	
Tools	
Temp	

	Carbs	Fat	Protein	Cals
Total				

KETO *Recipe*

RECIPE NAME:

_____

	Keto	Low Carb	Paleo	Vegetarian	Vegan	Dairy Free	Gluten Free
	☐	☐	☐	☐	☐	☐	☐

QTY	INGREDIENTS

RECIPE INSTRUCTIONS

NOTES & RECIPE REVIEW

Serves	
Prep Time	
Cook Time	
Tools	
Temp	

	Carbs	Fat	Protein	Cals
Total				

KETO *Recipe*

RECIPE NAME:

	Keto	Low Carb	Paleo	Vegetarian	Vegan	Dairy Free	Gluten Free
	☐	☐	☐	☐	☐	☐	☐

QTY	INGREDIENTS	RECIPE INSTRUCTIONS

NOTES & RECIPE REVIEW

Serves	
Prep Time	
Cook Time	
Tools	
Temp	

	Carbs	Fat	Protein	Cals
Total				

KETO *Recipe*

RECIPE NAME:

_____

	Keto	Low Carb	Paleo	Vegetarian	Vegan	Dairy Free	Gluten Free
	☐	☐	☐	☐	☐	☐	☐

QTY	INGREDIENTS

RECIPE INSTRUCTIONS

NOTES & RECIPE REVIEW

Serves	
Prep Time	
Cook Time	
Tools	
Temp	

	Carbs	Fat	Protein	Cals
Total				

KETO *Recipe*

RECIPE NAME:

	Keto	Low Carb	Paleo	Vegetarian	Vegan	Dairy Free	Gluten Free
	☐	☐	☐	☐	☐	☐	☐

QTY	INGREDIENTS	RECIPE INSTRUCTIONS

NOTES & RECIPE REVIEW

Serves	
Prep Time	
Cook Time	
Tools	
Temp	

	Carbs	Fat	Protein	Cals
Total				

KETO *Recipe*

RECIPE NAME:

_____

Keto	Low Carb	Paleo	Vegetarian	Vegan	Dairy Free	Gluten Free
☐	☐	☐	☐	☐	☐	☐

QTY	INGREDIENTS

RECIPE INSTRUCTIONS

NOTES & RECIPE REVIEW

Serves	
Prep Time	
Cook Time	
Tools	
Temp	

	Carbs	Fat	Protein	Cals
Total				

KETO *Recipe*

RECIPE NAME:

	Keto	Low Carb	Paleo	Vegetarian	Vegan	Dairy Free	Gluten Free
	☐	☐	☐	☐	☐	☐	☐

QTY	INGREDIENTS	RECIPE INSTRUCTIONS

NOTES & RECIPE REVIEW

Serves	
Prep Time	
Cook Time	
Tools	
Temp	

	Carbs	Fat	Protein	Cals
Total				

KETO *Recipe*

RECIPE NAME:

_____

Keto	Low Carb	Paleo	Vegetarian	Vegan	Dairy Free	Gluten Free
☐	☐	☐	☐	☐	☐	☐

QTY	INGREDIENTS

RECIPE INSTRUCTIONS

NOTES & RECIPE REVIEW

Serves	
Prep Time	
Cook Time	
Tools	
Temp	

	Carbs	Fat	Protein	Cals
Total				

KETO *Recipe*

RECIPE NAME:

	Keto	Low Carb	Paleo	Vegetarian	Vegan	Dairy Free	Gluten Free
	☐	☐	☐	☐	☐	☐	☐

QTY	INGREDIENTS	RECIPE INSTRUCTIONS

NOTES & RECIPE REVIEW

Serves	
Prep Time	
Cook Time	
Tools	
Temp	

	Carbs	Fat	Protein	Cals
Total				

KETO *Recipe*

RECIPE NAME:

Keto	Low Carb	Paleo	Vegetarian	Vegan	Dairy Free	Gluten Free
☐	☐	☐	☐	☐	☐	☐

QTY	INGREDIENTS

RECIPE INSTRUCTIONS

NOTES & RECIPE REVIEW

Serves	
Prep Time	
Cook Time	
Tools	
Temp	

	Carbs	Fat	Protein	Cals
Total				

KETO *Recipe*

RECIPE NAME:

	Keto	Low Carb	Paleo	Vegetarian	Vegan	Dairy Free	Gluten Free
	☐	☐	☐	☐	☐	☐	☐

QTY	INGREDIENTS	RECIPE INSTRUCTIONS

NOTES & RECIPE REVIEW	
Serves	
Prep Time	
Cook Time	
Tools	
Temp	

	Carbs	Fat	Protein	Cals
Total				

KETO *Recipe*

RECIPE NAME:

Keto	Low Carb	Paleo	Vegetarian	Vegan	Dairy Free	Gluten Free
☐	☐	☐	☐	☐	☐	☐

QTY	INGREDIENTS

RECIPE INSTRUCTIONS

NOTES & RECIPE REVIEW

Serves	
Prep Time	
Cook Time	
Tools	
Temp	

	Carbs	Fat	Protein	Cals
Total				

KETO *Recipe*

RECIPE NAME:

Keto	Low Carb	Paleo	Vegetarian	Vegan	Dairy Free	Gluten Free
☐	☐	☐	☐	☐	☐	☐

QTY	INGREDIENTS	RECIPE INSTRUCTIONS

NOTES & RECIPE REVIEW

Serves	
Prep Time	
Cook Time	
Tools	
Temp	

	Carbs	Fat	Protein	Cals
Total				

KETO *Recipe*

RECIPE NAME:
_____

	Keto	Low Carb	Paleo	Vegetarian	Vegan	Dairy Free	Gluten Free
	☐	☐	☐	☐	☐	☐	☐

QTY	INGREDIENTS

RECIPE INSTRUCTIONS

NOTES & RECIPE REVIEW

Serves	
Prep Time	
Cook Time	
Tools	
Temp	

	Carbs	Fat	Protein	Cals
Total				

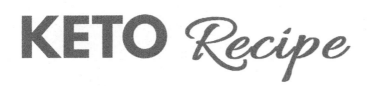

KETO *Recipe*

RECIPE NAME:

	Keto	Low Carb	Paleo	Vegetarian	Vegan	Dairy Free	Gluten Free
	☐	☐	☐	☐	☐	☐	☐

QTY	INGREDIENTS	RECIPE INSTRUCTIONS

NOTES & RECIPE REVIEW

Serves	
Prep Time	
Cook Time	
Tools	
Temp	

	Carbs	Fat	Protein	Cals
Total				

KETO *Recipe*

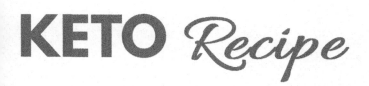

RECIPE NAME:

	Keto	Low Carb	Paleo	Vegetarian	Vegan	Dairy Free	Gluten Free
	☐	☐	☐	☐	☐	☐	☐

QTY	INGREDIENTS	RECIPE INSTRUCTIONS

NOTES & RECIPE REVIEW

Serves	
Prep Time	
Cook Time	
Tools	
Temp	

	Carbs	Fat	Protein	Cals
Total				

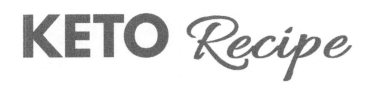

KETO *Recipe*

RECIPE NAME:

Keto ☐ Low Carb ☐ Paleo ☐ Vegetarian ☐ Vegan ☐ Dairy Free ☐ Gluten Free ☐

QTY	INGREDIENTS	RECIPE INSTRUCTIONS

NOTES & RECIPE REVIEW

Serves	
Prep Time	
Cook Time	
Tools	
Temp	

	Carbs	Fat	Protein	Cals
Total				

KETO *Recipe*

RECIPE NAME:

Keto	Low Carb	Paleo	Vegetarian	Vegan	Dairy Free	Gluten Free
☐	☐	☐	☐	☐	☐	☐

QTY	INGREDIENTS	RECIPE INSTRUCTIONS

NOTES & RECIPE REVIEW

Serves	
Prep Time	
Cook Time	
Tools	
Temp	

	Carbs	Fat	Protein	Cals
Total				

KETO *Recipe*

RECIPE NAME:

	Keto	Low Carb	Paleo	Vegetarian	Vegan	Dairy Free	Gluten Free
	☐	☐	☐	☐	☐	☐	☐

QTY	INGREDIENTS	RECIPE INSTRUCTIONS

NOTES & RECIPE REVIEW

Serves	
Prep Time	
Cook Time	
Tools	
Temp	

	Carbs	Fat	Protein	Cals
Total				

KETO *Recipe*

RECIPE NAME:

	Keto	Low Carb	Paleo	Vegetarian	Vegan	Dairy Free	Gluten Free
	☐	☐	☐	☐	☐	☐	☐

QTY	INGREDIENTS

RECIPE INSTRUCTIONS

NOTES & RECIPE REVIEW

Serves	
Prep Time	
Cook Time	
Tools	
Temp	

	Carbs	Fat	Protein	Cals
Total				

KETO *Recipe*

RECIPE NAME:

Keto ☐ Low Carb ☐ Paleo ☐ Vegetarian ☐ Vegan ☐ Dairy Free ☐ Gluten Free ☐

QTY	INGREDIENTS	RECIPE INSTRUCTIONS

NOTES & RECIPE REVIEW

Serves	
Prep Time	
Cook Time	
Tools	
Temp	

	Carbs	Fat	Protein	Cals
Total				

KETO *Recipe*

RECIPE NAME:

	Keto	Low Carb	Paleo	Vegetarian	Vegan	Dairy Free	Gluten Free
	☐	☐	☐	☐	☐	☐	☐

QTY	INGREDIENTS

RECIPE INSTRUCTIONS

NOTES & RECIPE REVIEW

Serves	
Prep Time	
Cook Time	
Tools	
Temp	

	Carbs	Fat	Protein	Cals
Total				

KETO *Recipe*

RECIPE NAME:

Keto	Low Carb	Paleo	Vegetarian	Vegan	Dairy Free	Gluten Free
☐	☐	☐	☐	☐	☐	☐

QTY	INGREDIENTS	RECIPE INSTRUCTIONS

NOTES & RECIPE REVIEW

Serves	
Prep Time	
Cook Time	
Tools	
Temp	

	Carbs	Fat	Protein	Cals
Total				

KETO *Recipe*

RECIPE NAME:

	Keto	Low Carb	Paleo	Vegetarian	Vegan	Dairy Free	Gluten Free
	☐	☐	☐	☐	☐	☐	☐

QTY	INGREDIENTS

RECIPE INSTRUCTIONS

NOTES & RECIPE REVIEW

Serves	
Prep Time	
Cook Time	
Tools	
Temp	

	Carbs	Fat	Protein	Cals
Total				

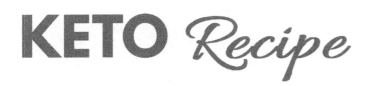

KETO *Recipe*

RECIPE NAME:

	Keto	Low Carb	Paleo	Vegetarian	Vegan	Dairy Free	Gluten Free
	☐	☐	☐	☐	☐	☐	☐

_____

QTY	INGREDIENTS	RECIPE INSTRUCTIONS

NOTES & RECIPE REVIEW

Serves	
Prep Time	
Cook Time	
Tools	
Temp	

	Carbs	Fat	Protein	Cals
Total				

KETO *Recipe*

RECIPE NAME:

	Keto	Low Carb	Paleo	Vegetarian	Vegan	Dairy Free	Gluten Free
	☐	☐	☐	☐	☐	☐	☐

QTY	INGREDIENTS

RECIPE INSTRUCTIONS

NOTES & RECIPE REVIEW

Serves	
Prep Time	
Cook Time	
Tools	
Temp	

	Carbs	Fat	Protein	Cals
Total				

KETO *Recipe*

RECIPE NAME:

_____

Keto	Low Carb	Paleo	Vegetarian	Vegan	Dairy Free	Gluten Free
☐	☐	☐	☐	☐	☐	☐

QTY	INGREDIENTS	RECIPE INSTRUCTIONS

NOTES & RECIPE REVIEW		Serves	
		Prep Time	
		Cook Time	
		Tools	
		Temp	

	Carbs	Fat	Protein	Cals
Total				

Made in the USA
Monee, IL
07 March 2021